BORROWED STORIES

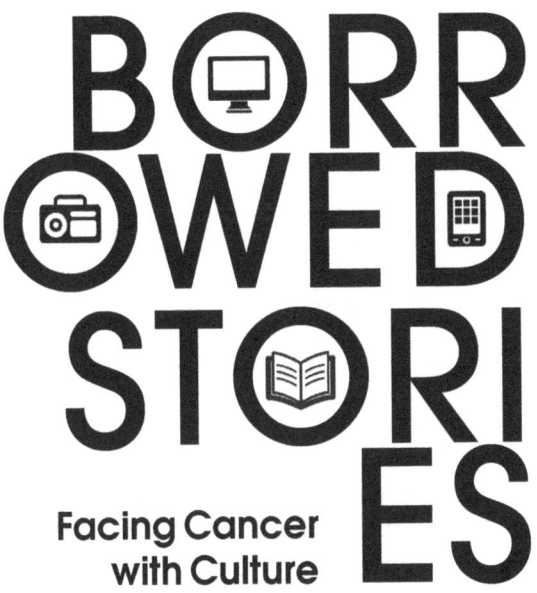

BORROWED STORIES

Facing Cancer with Culture from *Breaking Bad* to *The Divine Comedy*

EWAN BOWLBY

DARTON · LONGMAN + TODD
INTELLIGENT ♦ INSPIRATIONAL ♦ INCLUSIVE
SPIRITUAL BOOKS

First published in 2025 by
Darton, Longman and Todd Ltd
Unit 1, The Exchange
6 Scarbrook Road
Croydon CR0 1UH
editorial@darton-longman-todd.co.uk

This product conforms to the requirements of the European
Union's General Product Safety Regulations (GPSR).
EU Authorised Representative for GPSR:
Easy Access System Europe –
Mustamäe tee 50, 10621 Tallinn, Estonia
gpsr.requests@easproject.com

Complete text © 2025 Karlee Bowlby, with inclusion by licensed arrangement
of Editor's Note © 2025 Chris Bowlby
Foreword © 2025 Rowan Williams

The right of Ewan Bowlby to be identified as the Author of this work has been
asserted in accordance with the Copyright, Designs and Patents Act 1988.

ISBN: 978-1-917362-11-5

No part of this book may be used or reproduced in any manner for the
purpose of training artificial intelligence technologies or systems.

A catalogue record for this book is available from the British Library.

Printed and bound in Great Britain by Bell and Bain, Glasgow

CONTENTS

Foreword by Rowan Williams	7
Editor's Note by Chris Bowlby	10
Introduction	15
Part I	21
Chapter 1: Trading Stories	23
Chapter 2: Borrowed Stories	55
Part II	93
Chapter 1: Rethinking Spiritual Care	95
Chapter 2: Spiritual Care and the Arts	102
Chapter 3: Cancer, Time and Fiction	107
Chapter 4: Cancer, Paradox and *Breaking Bad*	129
Chapter 5: *The Bucket List*: Levity, Laughter and Living with Cancer	159
Chapter 6: Cancer, Emotion and Sentimentality	183
Final Thoughts	215
Postscript	217
Acknowledgements	219
Endnotes	221

FOREWORD BY ROWAN WILLIAMS

Where to begin with a book like this? Because in a way it's a book you might well wish had never had to be written, and yet that is precisely why it is a book that matters. The world is too full of shocking suffering and waste to do without a work of witness like this, a profoundly and persistently generous book in which the writer makes sense of what is happening by making a gift of his experience to those who might have to share it or something similar – or just those who need to know a bit more about living with dignity and vision through the end of a world.

Ewan was a genuine theological thinker in the academic context (I well remember animated conversation with him, and our shared delight at the intellect at work), but these pages show him as a theologian at another and different level. If we can talk about 'grace' here, it is not quite in the terms of traditional doctrine. It is something that comes through in the unplanned interruptions of insight, joy, urgency, immersion in the moment, all kinds of things that can't be systematized but insistently remind us of the truth that, if we're not in control of our living and dying, this can bring overwhelmingly good news as well as the opposite.

And at the same time, even while recognizing this lack of control, it is of the first importance to learn how to 'own' what is happening to you – not to let the experience be taken away and domesticated by institutional medicine, or institutional religion for that matter. Find what you need to tell your story and the people who will help you tell it. Don't be afraid of what it sounds like. Don't be afraid of saying what you need to make it really yours. If God is at work in all this, God wants you to be both a real created being, not fantasizing about being totally in charge of yourself, and a real creative being, making something new and unique out of it all.

The great Gillian Rose, one of the most outstanding philosophers of her generation, wrote in her last illness (in her late forties) of how she hoped to survive if only to become invisible and ordinary (like Miss Marple, she liked to say) – finding the skill just to be a skilled, compassionate, humorous part of the scenery, not a hero or a genius but a human being living truthfully. You might say – with some reason – that the world would be a much better place if that were indeed what being 'ordinary' meant. But you can see a bit what Gillian had in mind, and it is not too far from what Ewan had in mind. It's something to do with learning how to 'rest' in the potentially uncomfortable messiness of human experience, without the panicked effort to find the answer, the pattern. Which is why the arts become so important, not because they provide answers (they don't – or they provide too many and totally contradictory ones), but because they show how many different and chaotic things can, in spite of everything, be spoken about with honesty and insight. To be released from a false and limiting focus on 'objective' and scientific truth isn't to settle for a life of self-indulgent make-believe but to know how massive, elusive, and tantalizing a thing truth is. And for anyone who believes, that is rather what one might expect in a world that depends on and is pervaded by an elusive but never-absent 'accompanier', the God who is witness and lover and enigma and goal all at once.

All of this Ewan says far better (and sharper and funnier) than I can. Tragic that a young man of exceptional gifts should have to write such a book? Well, yes and no. Nothing takes the loss away or makes it anything but what it is. But that loss brings a gift, not one that anyone would ever choose at the hand of someone they love, yet perhaps the only thing that makes the loss capable of being lived with; a new depth of resource for others to find how to tell their story; a new opening up of the possibility of grace.

RW

EDITOR'S NOTE BY CHRIS BOWLBY

When our son Ewan Bowlby was diagnosed with a brain tumour at the age of 17, he might have been expected to spend as much time as possible trying to distract himself from the implications. In the last decade of his life, he moved instead in a very different direction. He chose to devote himself fully to exploring his own experience and that of other cancer sufferers. He worked at the top level academically, but what he wanted above all was for his insights and work to spread as far as possible and help others facing what he had to face. This book – a combination of Ewan's personal story and his ideas about improving care for everyone – aims to fulfil that ambition.

His own perspective was unique but shaped by an unusually interesting range of family and other influences, defying all the usual labels. Theology was his formal field of academic study – an interest sparked partly by one of his grandfathers, Bishop Ronnie Bowlby. But Ronnie's and Ewan's idea of theology, or the 'spiritual', was never about dogma or abstract debate. It was about helping people face whatever they had to, including the most fundamental 'big questions' of life, and death.

EDITOR'S NOTE BY CHRIS BOWLBY

Ewan linked those interests in his work to another area – culture. Again, this might suggest a restricted focus on more highbrow interests. But Ewan's other grandfather, and another great influence, was the poet Tony Harrison. He encouraged an interest in the cultural life of all kinds of communities, and the ability of the arts to help confront every kind of human experience, including the darkest. One of my clearest early memories of Ewan is his rapt absorption as a five-year-old in the wonderful drama of Tony's version of the medieval mystery plays at the National Theatre.

As his work shows, Ewan always moved easily between what some might see as 'high' and 'low' culture. One of our great bonds was supporting, for our sins, Newcastle United. Sometimes, faced with the team's latest failure, I would apologise for having led him into this. He proudly replied that, on the contrary, he had benefited as supporting them had 'taught me everything I need to know about existential despair'. Humour – everything from joyous hilarity to a sharp sense of irony – was, as you will see in chapter 5 of the second part of this book, one of Ewan's favourite responses to what he experienced and had to endure.

After studying at Cambridge, writing a dissertation on Dostoevsky supervised by Rowan Williams, Ewan found a new home well suited to his interests at the University of St Andrews in the Institute for Theology, Imagination and the Arts. But academia was never enough. He might sit in an academic seminar one morning, and then get on a bus to Dundee to talk to a beloved support group of fellow cancer sufferers from all walks of life in the afternoon. And his work, as you will see, happily ranged from Dostoevsky and Dante to the latest hit TV drama.

Ewan died at the end of 2022. It was the final extreme rollercoaster of a year for us in a decade of living with his brain tumour and then cancer. That summer, we had the family celebration of his marriage to Karlee, a fellow student at St Andrews. A few months later, he and we had the shattering experience of going into a room for the results of his latest brain scan, where his oncologist explained that his cancer, now a glioblastoma, was spreading rapidly and he had at most a few months to live. There was of course despair for all of us. But Ewan being Ewan, there was also a desire to make the best even of this most awful of situations.

He managed to reach one landmark in his work when St Andrews accelerated the assessment of his PhD. He was awarded the doctorate in a virtual ceremony which we showed him on a laptop as he lay, increasingly weak, in bed in his flat near to us in Northumberland.

But he had always wanted to produce another kind of work, much more personal. Ewan was very keen that his thoughts on the way in which the arts and popular culture can help patients would reach a wider audience well beyond the academic world. He had begun to write this in the form of two autobiographical chapters, the first two chapters in what follows. In them, Ewan describes how his illness affected him and how he came to understand the need to talk about it as his story, but a story that could help others too – not only those who suffer from cancer or other severe illnesses, but all those who care for them personally and professionally.

The rest of the book was going to be based loosely on his doctorate. His plan had been to turn the PhD, freed from some of its more formal style and strict presentational rules, into a 'popular' publication.

But then, cruelly, his time ran out. When Ewan knew that was happening, we talked about what could be done, how the story could still be told – and he asked me to take on the task of adapting his thesis for that wider audience. As he explains in the first chapter, throughout the previous decade we and his mum Jane had often talked with him about how to make sense of all that he was going through, and how it related to other things our family had experienced. We now had the most moving but also practical conversations about the legacy he wanted to leave. 'That was a helpful and exciting chat earlier' he messaged me after one conversation. 'I'm really glad to be leaving the book in your safe hands'.

I remember reading that message with a mixture of feelings so typical of those months before he died: daunted and grief-stricken at having to take on such a task, yet honoured and, as so often in Ewan's short life, immensely proud of the way he responded to what fate had thrown at him.

So, after Ewan's first two chapters, what follows is based on his academic work, which is available online as a formal PhD. Anyone who wants to discover all the details of the research he did and the authors he consulted can find it fully referenced there. What I have tried to do here, as he asked me to do, is keep close to Ewan's argument and voice, but create something more direct and most focused on the people he encountered rather than external sources.

Part II is based on the structure of his thesis and retains most of his language. The style of these chapters remains more formal than the two personal chapters in Part I, but the argument is no less heartfelt. In preparing them, in the spirit of my conversations with Ewan, I have tried to keep his argument as clear as possible while removing some of the material and language that was aimed more at satisfying formal requirements or engaging in academic debate, rather than central to what he wanted to offer the wider world.

In a few places, I have added short passages where I felt this would offer context, help the flow and highlight the main points. Rather than footnotes within the text, a list of the sources referenced is included as endnotes at the end of the book.

None of this is intended in any way to downplay the contributions of all those whose work helped shape Ewan's academic understanding; and I am delighted that his doctorate is available too for those who want to follow that side of things. But I hope all will understand the commitment we feel to fulfilling Ewan's wish – that his work be available and influential in different ways.

The personal introduction to his work Ewan had been writing finishes on, for him, a characteristic note of 'perseverance, resilience and hope'. That is what carried him through an extraordinary decade in which he lived such a rich, creative life despite what was hanging over him after his first diagnosis. When he had lost hope for his own survival, he could still express with passion another kind of hope – that what he had experienced, researched and articulated could live on and bring to as many people as possible some of the insights and benefits that he, in his brilliantly courageous way, had discovered.

CB

INTRODUCTION

'IF HIS NEXT SCAN shows progression then this would be much more concerning and it might be that his prognosis is measured in months. But if his next scan is stable or better it could perhaps be short years'. Told in blunt medical language, this is the story of the brain cancer that will end my life. Taken from a recent letter from my oncologist, these words explain that my life is fragile and uncertain, its length dependent on the success of treatment. I am twenty-seven years old, and I have an aggressive, cancerous tumour in my brain. This situation is the culmination of ten years of living with a brain tumour; while it began as a benign lump of cells, over time the tumour has evolved into a lethal cancer. This gradual progression has given me time to develop a relationship with death, learning to respect and accept the presence of death in my life. I have spent years thinking, writing and talking about death and disease, searching for ways of approaching mortality with clarity, honesty and creativity. Although seeking out a more intimate relationship with human transience might seem a macabre, unhealthy obsession, this work has been vital for my soul. My devoted study of the emotional, existential impact of terminal illness has helped me to tell a new story about myself and my approaching death. This is a richer, deeper and more meaningful story than my medical documents can tell. It is not just about the medical fight against disease, doing everything possible to prolong my life whatever the cost; it is a story about love, care and dependence. Learning to tell this story has helped me to embrace honesty and vulnerability, recognising my reliance on those who support me instead of trying to solve the problem of death on my own. My hope is that by using my remaining life to tell people how I found my story, I might help others threatened by death to discover their own stories and find new meaning in their lives.

I want to tell this story because, for those close to death, many people believe the situation is hopeless – devoid of either the chance of recovering or of making peace with a life cut short. They tell us that we are a society in 'denial of death', incapable of accepting our mortality. The idea of 'the denial of death' was popularised by the American cultural anthropologist Ernst Becker. Becker believed that we have, unconsciously, designed human civilisation to distract us from our 'helplessness and terror' when faced with death, creating mythologies and symbols that allow us to believe that we can somehow transcend mortality. Becker also argued that, with the decline of religious belief in Western society, we have lost one of the most important 'illusions' that eased our death anxiety. Since then, his warnings about our fear of death, and the loss of the 'systems' and stories that can address this fear, have been echoed by many other scholars and social commentators. While the bleak pessimism of these claims about our collective denial of death can be alluring, I want to use my story to present a more hopeful perspective. Such dire warnings about our inadequate cultural resources and collective terror are powerful, but I believe that they go too far. It is important

INTRODUCTION

to draw attention to our difficulties when it comes to death and disease, but we must not overlook the sources of hope, inspiration and consolation that are available to us. My suspicion is that those making drastic statements about our denial of death have failed to look in unexpected places for the cultural and social resources that they claim are entirely absent in the contemporary Western world. In this book, I describe how I found inspiring, revealing storytelling about death in a wide range of places: Netflix, young adult novels, Hollywood films, local support groups, sitcoms, hospital waiting rooms. These are places that those denouncing our lack of cultural and social tools for dealing with death and disease do not seem to have looked. Many times, I have come across words, ideas and examples that helped me to tell my story in areas of our lives that rarely feature in grandiose discussions of the denial of death. Although we may have lost sight of the forms of meaning and consolation that religion used to offer to the sick and dying, I believe that there are still many examples today of people using art, imagination and creativity to find meaning in mortality. And I do not think that these are merely offering what Becker calls 'illusions': tricks designed to help us maintain our denial of death. I believe that many people in modern society are confronting mortality with honesty, bravery and ingenuity.

My aim is to draw attention to some of the things that have helped me to find meaning: the 'tools' that enabled me to move from denial to acceptance. As the title of this book suggests, it has only been by borrowing from other stories that I have learned to tell my own cancer story, speaking openly about my illness and approaching death. The idea of 'borrowed stories', itself borrowed from cancer patient and sociologist Arthur Frank, helps me to explain how I have relied on hearing real and fictional stories to find my own voice as a storyteller. Every ill person has a unique story, and many aspects of each distinct narrative will not be relevant to others trying to come to terms with their mortality. But my hope is that at least some elements of my story will prove resonant for anyone who is seeking new perspectives on disease and death. Even when my experiences seem entirely alien to another person, a strong negative reaction could also prove revealing for their search for meaning. We learn from what repels us, discovering more about our own desires and inclinations when this happens. In an attempt to make this book as valuable as possible, I have chosen to focus on four themes that I believe will seem relevant and important to anyone who has had a serious illness: time, death, humour and relationship. I am eager to pass on the wisdom and insight that I have benefited from: the ideas and stories of fellow patients that have taught me so much about myself. Hearing the ways that people affected by cancer respond to fictional stories about their disease is fascinating, revealing and rewarding, and this book seeks to extend this opportunity to readers.

However, in Part I, I begin this book by telling the unique, personal story of my illness. This seems a natural starting point, as this book is about how I overcame crippling anxiety and incoherency so that I could tell others about my cancer. It also allows me to offer my own story as something that others can borrow from, adopting my words in order to interpret or speak about their own experiences of illness. However, this is complicated by the fact that my story is still unfolding. It may be drawing close to its conclusion, but new chapters are still being added. In fact, it has recently started to resemble a love story, its course and colours changing as it assumes new shades of joy, romance, and possibility. The uncertainty and unpredictability of my

INTRODUCTION

condition means that this project stands on shifting sands, as it is repeatedly rendered outdated by new developments in my situation. Writing this book is further complicated by my fragile, unstable health. I am currently recovering from brain surgery, chemotherapy, and radiation treatment. Earlier this year, I learned that my brain cancer had returned in a more aggressive form. Following urgent surgery, a course of chemotherapy was used to target any remaining cancer cells. But as anyone familiar with chemotherapy will know, this is not a subtle method of treatment. Cytotoxic chemotherapy drugs disrupt and destroy cancer cells, but they also harm other cells, causing indiscriminate damage to a patient's body. The radiotherapy treatment that followed also causes collateral damage, further weakening and harming my body and brain.

Consequently, my energy, attention and creative capacities are limited. Extreme fatigue, alongside a strange and unpredictable array of side effects caused by surgery, toxicity and radiation continue to trouble me. Such bodily and psychological scarring takes time to heal and, as I have learned, its impact can linger. Even the physical effort of drafting this book, dragging pen across paper, is sometimes more than I'm capable of.

My memory is also unreliable. When my cancer was first diagnosed six years ago, I underwent seven weeks of radiotherapy treatment. The harm caused by having radiation fired at the brain daily for this length of time is something that still hinders me. It is common for this collateral damage to cause permanent memory problems, and this is what I have experienced. Recently, after the cancer returned in a more deadly form, I had to undergo 'repeat radiotherapy', with radiation targeted again at the same area of the brain. This brings increased risks, with the possibility of brain 'necrosis' (healthy brain cells in the irradiated area dying). The likelihood of serious memory problems, confusion and mental disability also increases each time radiation is used on the brain. Clinicians have also suggested that the tumour itself may have affected my decision-making and memory. The overall effect of this is that my intellect is unsteady and hesitant, perhaps ill-equipped to try to convey ideas with eloquence and precision. I cannot promise to be able to relate past events with exacting accuracy, and I must ask readers to be forgiving if the focus or clarity of the prose slips on occasion. I have a dilapidated, weary brain, and I have no choice but to write out of this position of neurodiversity and neurovulnerability. In place of accuracy, consistency and lucidity, I offer authenticity and honesty.

It is the moments of drama and emotional intensity that have settled best in my memory: vivid and detailed pictures that I can still call to mind without difficulty. So, I can write with confidence about the times that I have experienced powerful feelings of grief, despair, pain, joy, or hope. I can describe these pivotal points in my story, and I hope this will be enough. I also hope that it might be interesting to read this attempt to tell my story precisely because it emerges out of my struggles with weakness and fatigue. My position of vulnerability and dependence seems a good starting point for this project, as it is about my reliance on other people and the meaning they add to my life. It is a book about borrowing; about how we cannot search for meaning alone but must look for the rich resources that fellow humans offer us as we face our mortality.

PART I

PART I

Chapter 1
TRADING STORIES

When, at the age of twenty-one, I was diagnosed with incurable brain cancer, I discovered how serious illness changes our life story. Following a diagnosis like this, the ways that we previously understood ourselves and our situation no longer make sense. Cancer patients often find that questions like 'How are you?', or even 'Who are you?', become very difficult to answer; a life that may once have seemed like a gradual journey towards a clear destination can be disrupted by the physical and psychological roadblock of cancer. Medical sociologist Arthur Frank describes this as the 'loss of a destination and map' caused by serious illness. Faced with cancer, we can lose sight of where we are going and how we're getting there, and that is what I experienced.

The story of the cancer that will end my life began when I was sixteen years old. While playing football with my father I collapsed and had a seizure. I was rushed to hospital in an ambulance. At a later appointment, a doctor decided that what had happened to me was a 'vasovagal syncope'; in other words, he thought I had fainted. It is telling that I accepted this unquestioningly. At this point, the story I told about myself was still that of a sporty, active, 'normal' teenage boy who was in good health. But over the next nine months my faith in this story was gradually eroded. The seizures kept happening, and I regularly found myself in hospital having collapsed.

These seizures happened in many different places: at home, playing football, overnight in bed. The second, and perhaps most difficult time came when I had a seizure in the school playground. I had been enjoying a game of football with friends, then lost consciousness before waking up with a paramedic standing over me. I later discovered that the seizure happened at the end of break time, so that hundreds of my fellow students had returned to the classrooms adjacent to the playground in time to watch me shaking, violently and uncontrollably, on the tarmac. Then, they watched an ambulance drive into the playground and unload the paramedics that came to take me to hospital. In retrospect, I have recognised this as a moment in which my story began to change irrevocably. Friends later told me that they had thought, while the seizure was happening, that they were watching me die. For most of the school, this was the point at which I came to be uniquely associated with vulnerability and mortality. I was the person responsible for an ambulance – the vivid, foreboding *memento mori* of modern society – intruding into a community of young men for whom death and disease were still abstract, distant concepts.

Many more seizures followed, and with them came a swelling sense of unease, a burgeoning awareness that something was seriously wrong in my body. My illusions of youthful vigour and invincibility were further undermined with each of these inexplicable episodes. Doctors began a frantic search for something to rectify: an exhaustive probing of my heart, lungs, blood pressure, liver. All of this contributed to my awareness of a nameless, mysterious threat to my safety and wellbeing. Although my recollections of this period are patchy and unreliable, I can remember vividly the sensation that always preceded a seizure. I would suddenly be gripped by a feeling of heavy, dragging inevitability: a realisation that I had lost control of my body. The helplessness and fear that accompanied this realisation came to define this time for me. Seizure after seizure added to my suspicions that my life was beginning to spiral, dizzyingly, knocking me off course. Eventually, my body found a more persuasive, powerful way of drawing attention to a profound problem. One morning, while putting on my school shoes, I was overcome with nausea and exhaustion, left too unwell to move. My mother took me to our local doctor, who glanced at me once before telling her to take me straight to the hospital.

My next clear memory is of waking in a hospital ward in which all the other inhabitants were elderly men. My memories after that comprise sporadic spells of wakefulness during which I heard, ceaselessly, cries of discomfort, distress or confusion. I found myself in the midst of the care crisis of our times: beds full of people in old age, left frail and disorientated by suffering, slipping towards death as their life force is crushed beneath the weight of chronic illness. I cannot claim to have found any sense of solidarity with these aged patients at the time; my capacity for feelings of companionship with patients much older than me had not yet developed. But I do believe that the experience of sharing a space with a group of men who had passed the point at which our society welcomes and accommodates them, having become too redolent of death, was sufficiently humbling to prepare me for what came next.

When I eventually returned to full consciousness, I had been moved to a private ward. And in this ward, my story changed direction again. With no warning – no gentle, careful preamble – a consultant came into my room and began to speak about a brain tumour. She had not been aware that the possibility of a brain tumour had not yet been raised, so that this was the first time I was confronted with the idea. But this encounter was, to a certain extent, characteristic of a healthcare system that has come to prioritise curing over communication. Working with dwindling resources in increasingly challenging conditions, it is perfectly reasonable for healthcare professionals to put saving lives ahead of salving souls. This was the first time I learned about the human consequences of a culture of time-pressure and 'efficiency' drives, in which the way disease and diagnosis are talked about appears relatively unimportant. It was also the first time I had to entertain the idea of something unwanted and potentially lethal lurking in my brain.

That this idea arrived in my consciousness so abruptly only added to its impact. The way this affected my mind, at the age of seventeen, was analogous to the tumour itself, a dense mass of troubling thoughts. During that brief conversation with a clinician, something took root in my imagination: a dark, impenetrable obstacle that could not be seen into or past. After the initial shock of hearing the word tumour, the darkness started to spread from this mass, disrupting and infecting other areas of my consciousness. Planning, anticipating and preparing became far more complex than they had been before. My visions of the future now seemed fragile and contingent, and my capacity for unalloyed joy, simply resting in calm enjoyment of the present, was also diminished.

Soon, I was attending meetings with strangers who seemed to hold my fate in their hands. These new characters in my story: neurologists, oncologists, surgeons, were – from the outset – central figures. Normally, for a person to become a significant part of my life took time. Friendship and romance were about inching tentatively towards intimacy, trust and mutual dependence. But I soon realised that I would have to learn to trust clinicians and place my faith in them from our first meeting. I would walk into a consultation room, shake hands with someone I had never met before, and a few minutes later we would be discussing the prospect of a brain tumour ending my life. After a series of these bizarre encounters, which usually ended with a referral to another consultant, I found myself in a meeting with a surgeon. Somewhere along the way it had been decided that a craniotomy (brain surgery) was necessary for 'debulking' (reducing the size of the tumour). The tumour was still, at this point, grade two; in other words, it was benign and not cancerous. Oncologists and surgeons talk about 'grades' of brain tumour as a way of conveying how dangerous each tumour is, and how it is likely to behave. I suspect that this may be, in part, a way of avoiding calling something cancer (more on that subject later). My team of consultants saw surgery as the best option because it would reduce the chances of seizures and make it less likely that the tumour would change from grade two to grade three: a more aggressive, dangerous form.

There is a kind of gravity to the phrase 'brain surgery'. For many people, it evokes awe and terror. But, in the end, I found it to be an anti-climactic experience. Thanks to the strange magic of general anaesthetic, there was relatively little suffering involved. I remember being sent to sleep then waking up what felt like seconds later in a recovery ward. Because of the drugs and painkillers, I was high when I did regain consciousness, which only added to the impression that I had undergone a trivial, straightforward procedure. My mother was allowed to join me in the recovery room and later told me – to my intense embarrassment – that she found me flirting outrageously with the nurses. That I had the energy and confidence for that testifies to the elation and relief that I felt once the surgery was successfully completed.

It was only once the high wore off that I noticed the signs of what had happened to me. Nausea, pain and fatigue arrived. I have since come to know these three old friends intimately, but the first seventeen years of my life had been blissfully free of their unwelcome presence, so this was a shock. Then, I saw the scar. The sight of a bandage scarcely concealing a red, inflamed slash across my forehead was a visible, tangible token left by the surgical team that made it impossible to doubt what had happened to me. Seeing that, I had to begin to work out how to reconcile myself to the idea of a group of strangers spending hours cutting, sawing and exploring inside my skull. This was the first time that I experienced the unsettling effects of the gap general anaesthetic creates in your life. It was as if my story had been gradually building towards a key event only for a blank page to appear at the crucial moment. Then, the narrative begins again with me scarred and unwell, leaving a clear sense that something significant had happened, but also a disconcerting lack of detail.

I have realised, having heard others talk about similar experiences, that this strange gap affected my ability to process what had happened. Having surgery under general anaesthetic is like flying to another country. You arrive at the airport, go through the preparatory stages, and board the plane. Then, in a few hours, you disembark in a radically different place with a climate and landscape that are unfamiliar. By contrast, if you take the train instead, you have a long time to acclimatise; you see gradual changes in the plants, buildings and weather. By the time you eventually arrive, your mind and body have had an opportunity to adjust. Whilst I would later discover that the surgical equivalent to taking the train is profoundly unpleasant (an awake craniotomy: more on that later), the abrupt arrival in a daunting place when you wake from general anaesthetic is disconcerting. The mismatch between the scarring and trauma that the eye sees and body feels and the blank absence in what the mind recalls is jarring.

This tension was one of the factors that contributed to my difficulties as I tried to come to terms with my new role as an Ill Person. The scar was an indelible mark that made it difficult to ignore the fact that a new chapter had begun in my story. Yet ignoring this was exactly what I tried to do. I continued to try to live the life of a lively seventeen-year-old boy by playing sport, partying, studying for exams and chasing girls. This was not a conscious, considered decision. In fact, I was not even aware that by carrying on as if nothing had changed, I was making a choice. It simply did not occur to me that I might have needed to set aside some time to process and heal, and to reappraise my situation. I did not pause to notice that my story was changing. At this point, dying of cancer remained an abstract, distant possibility. When my tumour was diagnosed, relatively little was known about how it might behave in the future. I was told that it could change into a more dangerous 'grade three' tumour if left untreated, becoming something that was a threat to life. But when this might happen, and the likelihood of it ever happening, were presented as unknowns. Given the lack of data and clinical certainty surrounding brain tumours at the time, this was entirely reasonable. Reticence and caution are surely appropriate when speaking to a teenager about something lodged in their brain that could, one day, end their life. Yet these tentative, brief allusions to the prospect of death were enough to place an anxiety in the depths of my consciousness.

Rather than bringing this new anxiety, and the inner tumult it set in motion, into the light, I opted to leave it buried. Again, this was not an active choice. I did not have the powers of emotional expression to name or describe the hidden, interiorised fear and instability that the allusions to death caused. Death had yet to feature in any real, tangible way in my story, and I was still developing and maturing, learning about the kinds of vulnerability and honesty required for meaningful human interaction. I would not have known how to go about asking for help, and my range of options still seemed limited to only those things that I could achieve independently. I was surrounded by caring, wise family members and good friends, but I didn't realise that I needed their help. So, instead of seeking support and beginning to try to process my condition, I threw myself back into my everyday existence as if nothing had changed. I was academically ambitious and had always intended to apply to a prestigious university. That necessitated intensive study as I sat a series of exams that would determine the direction my education took. At the time, I believed my performance in exams would determine the course of my life; I had not yet found the healthy dose of perspective that a life-threatening illness can bring. So, I continued to devote time and energy to cramming facts, ideas and exam tips into my memory, leaving limited space for my mind to deal with other things. The feverish, frantic nature of revising under self-imposed pressure was only exacerbated by the complications of enforced breaks and fatigue caused by brain surgery.

Once I had recovered from the surgery, I soon reverted to seeking release in sport and socialising. The thrill and camaraderie of team sports, particularly football, had for most of my childhood been a nourishing, uplifting part of my life. I wanted to continue to tell myself and others the story of an athletic, healthy young man sharing the fun of sporting contests with my peers. The only change to this story that I had to acknowledge was the head guard that I needed to wear while playing football to protect the area of my skull weakened by surgery. This 'scrum cap', a type of headgear more usually worn by rugby players, was the one sign betraying my changed situation that I could not conceal. And because it did not belong on a football pitch, it made me a target for mockery. Opposition players rarely managed to think of anything more creative than shouting 'Petr Čech' at me (the name of a famous footballer who also had to wear a scrum cap, due to a serious head injury). In fact, it made for a refreshing change when one more inventive opponent told me that I 'looked like a condom' while wearing the cap. Despite the monotony and predictability of the taunts, they were painful. I am sure it never occurred to any of my abusers that I was wearing the cap as the legacy of brain surgery. But this was still my first experience of the ways that illness can mark you out, set you apart, and make you feel lonely while surrounded by people. It may also have been one of the first experiences that made me aware of the fact that there was another story running parallel to my old one, undermining a more conventional narrative. Over time, I would become increasingly conscious of the tensions between these two stories, but I was not yet ready to contemplate surrendering the familiar life story that I had grown up with.

Ignoring these tensions became much more difficult

when I had to undergo brain surgery a second time. Scans had revealed that the tumour was growing again, and because leaving a large tumour unchecked risked it becoming cancerous, my surgeon was keen to act. This news shattered any illusions of the first operation being an isolated event. I could no longer try to pretend that my condition was something that could be resolved with a single procedure. Rather than living through brain surgery, I found myself living with a brain tumour. This shift in perspective meant the psychological impact was greater the second time around, and the disruption caused was also more significant. I was on the cusp of the exams and interviews that would determine the next phase of my education. The success of my university applications was dependent on high grades in my final exams, and the unexpected difficulties that more surgery would cause seemed an intolerable threat to my aspirations. Trying to revise and give a good account of myself in an interview while recovering from brain surgery was a grim prospect. There was already a sense of pressure as my intellect and focus wavered under the weight of self-imposed expectations, and to put my brain through the trauma of surgery again would, I believed, only add to this burden. Despite this, my instinct was still to fight to hold onto the original life story that I imagined for myself. I never contemplated adapting my plans, reshaping my vision for the future to fit around the intrusion of serious illness. I have no doubt that, had I shown any inclination to make room for respite and recovery, those caring for me would have welcomed and affirmed my decision. But I was not ready to entertain the idea of rethinking my story. Looking back, I find it difficult not to sympathise with my seventeen-year-old self. My life experience had not yet taught me to see all life plans as contingent, dependent on naïve assumptions about the smooth predictability and consistency of human existence. Before painful lessons are learned, it seems understandable and natural that we follow our youthful inclination to pursue dreams single-mindedly and relentlessly.

And that is what I did. Once again, the surgery was successful and uneventful. Five hours were neatly excised from my conscious life by general anaesthetic, and I woke with nausea, a headache and a more pronounced scar. The only moment of jeopardy came before the surgery when I arrived at the hospital. I was greeted with the news that there may not be a bed available after the surgery, so the procedure might need to be postponed. In recent years, so many patients have experienced the deflating disappointment of preparing, bracing for surgery, only to learn it must be delayed. For some hours, I found myself in this position, uncertain as to whether the operation that I had been anticipating for weeks could go ahead. Since spending time in that liminal, awful position, I have always held the deepest sympathy for those who have had surgery delayed because it was not deemed sufficiently urgent. Enduring the fierce apprehension that inevitably precedes surgery only to have to find a way to release such strong emotion must be profoundly disheartening. In the end, the severity of my condition and my youth worked in my favour, and a bed was somehow found. This was the first of many times in my cancer story that I was given cause to consider other patients who had been deprioritised. Every time that a bed is found, a scan fitted in, or an urgent operation scheduled, someone else suffers. I had become a priority in a healthcare system in which decisions must constantly be made about whose need is greatest because of a paucity of resources, time and space. You are aware that your illness is often weighed against others to determine who should take precedence, coming to understand that there is a human cost every time you are treated as an urgent case demanding swift action. So, I am grateful for the anxious moment in which I briefly experienced what it is like to discover that plans for your treatment are vulnerable to the pressures of the NHS; since then, whenever a clinician has intervened to 'squeeze me in' I have offered a silent prayer for the other patients that pay the price.

Eventually, after some frantic searching by my surgical team, a bed was found. The surgery went ahead and was successful. Because of my young age, I was given a private room, separate from the adult neurology ward around me, to recover in. I was grateful for the relative peace and privacy this afforded me. It also made it easier for friends and family to visit, providing a continued connection to the security, companionship and familiarity of the outside world. But, since then, I have wondered whether this instinct to set younger patients apart, screening them from the realities of disease, infirmity and senility, is a good thing. As I will explain later, honesty and friendship shared with people further down the path of life has been vital in my movement towards a healthy relationship with death. And this intentional separation from other, older people navigating serious illness deprived me of an opportunity to learn from fellow patients. This separation may also have encouraged me to internalise further a desire to distance myself from the unvarnished truth of death and disease, to continue to see myself as somehow unconnected to decaying and dying. This special treatment reinforced the notion that it was unnatural or unacceptable for a teenager to be living close to death.

Recovering while cut off from the bustle and drama of the main ward also made it easier for me to treat the second round of surgery as an irritating, insignificant distraction from the serious business of living my life. I continued to follow a familiar path, forcing my story to play out in the way I desired and expected. A few weeks after the operation, I returned to intense revision for exams. This was supplemented by regular parties, as several friends celebrated their eighteenth birthdays. My parents, understandably concerned, urged rest and caution but the only course of action I could conceive was a full-blooded return to my previous way of life. I did not pause for long enough to ask myself, let alone to ask others, about what the implications of the tumour in my brain might be. I could not entertain the possibility of my story beginning to move in a different direction, of a new 'destination and map' that took into account my condition. Rather than pause to catch my breath, think, talk and process, I charged forwards. There is, admittedly, very little room in the whorl of exams, applications and interviews for young people in education to find moments for calm reflection. But even if such an opportunity had presented itself, I would not have known how to use it.

In the end, it seemed that my decision to press ahead with university applications and prior plans was justified. To my surprise and delight, I was offered a place at Cambridge University to study theology. Then, I somehow scraped together the grades that I needed to meet the conditions of my offer. I remember the summer holiday after I finally finished those exams as a time of blissful release as the stress and exhaustion that had accumulated dissipated. I threw myself into celebrating, drunk on freedom and relief (and, sometimes, alcohol). One of the things contributing to this feeling was a belief that my story was back on track; I had secured the future that I had always aimed at and

I was feeling lively, young and healthy again. The hole in my cerebral cortex, where a tumour had once been, did not feature prominently in my thoughts. Amongst the many sources of fun and excitement that distracted from this hole was the arrival of romance in my story. During my final years at school, I had grown close to a kind, attractive girl who had been particularly caring and attentive while I struggled with my health.

Caught up in the paradise of a summer without exams or studying, we became a couple. My relationship with Kate, who proved to be a patient, sympathetic and compassionate partner, became a crucial part of my story. But as we fell in love, I did not consider how my tumour – which I knew could return at any time – might affect our relationship. From an early stage, we were discussing a shared future and family. I had been told by clinicians several times that my tumour could never be definitively 'cured', so the risk of recurrence would always remain. The threat of the tumour returning in a cancerous, dangerous form was something I would always carry with me. But I still treated this as a truth only loosely, tangentially connected to my main storyline. In the rapture of first love, indulging in daydreams is irresistible, and an idyllic future life with Kate began to take shape in my imagination.

But more important than this was the emotional support and companionship that Kate provided during my first few years as a student. Throughout my childhood, and especially once I became ill, my family home had been the place where I felt secure, loved and confident. My miraculous, precious parents and siblings (who I will return to later), were a reliable source of joy, peace and support. The extent to which I had been dependent on my family while I was unwell only became clear once I left home to go to university. Initially, I embraced the new social and intellectual challenges of university life, making new friends and getting to grips with a different mode of learning. But after my first term I found myself beset by intense feelings of loneliness, anxiety and fatigue. A Cambridge year is structured around short, sharp bursts of learning and essay-writing, demanding hours of rigorous study every day. The pressures that this placed on me, when combined with navigating an unfamiliar social scene and separation from family life, proved to be more than I was able to manage. The exhaustion and apprehension that I had not addressed or acknowledged while going through sickness, seizures and surgery finally came to the surface. When these powerful feelings were exacerbated by the routines of Cambridge life, mingling with the stress and isolation I experienced, I was no longer able to suppress or conceal my buried emotions.

During my first year, I became progressively more burdened with dark, unsettling thoughts and feelings. I lost all desire to spend time with other students, and the university nightlife lost its appeal. Without the reassurance of family nearby, I felt lost. One day, shortly before the Christmas holidays, I found myself alone in my student accommodation, weeping. I had just been given another assignment to complete over the break and the mounting pile of books that I had to read, digest and write about over the festive season had broken my spirit. Because of the strength of the desperation I felt, my memory of that moment is still keen. I was overtaken by a helplessness that was alien to me. The sense of being unable to rely on my own resources, of defeat and utter exhaustion, was not something I had experienced before. It did not fit with my story of a capable, independent, strong young man, who could take new challenges in his stride. My descent into helplessness also challenged the 'restitution narrative' of modern medicine, where a patient is treated, cured, and sent out into the world as a healthy, rejuvenated person. Subconsciously, I had bought into this attractive narrative, rather than anticipating further complications to my health. So, the unfamiliar incapacity and vulnerability that I was experiencing were undermining a reassuring, neat story in which my illness had been decisively dealt with. I had heard the warnings about my tumour returning, but nobody had ever discussed the long-term legacy of serious illness and surgery: the emotional and physical impact that continues long after treatment is finished.

We tend to think of scarring as purely physical; we picture scars as the outwardly visible, tangible signs of bodily injury. Yet what I was affected by as an undergraduate was mental, spiritual scarring. Two years of medical drama had caused forms of internal, hidden damage, leaving me with a bruised, tender soul and a fragile mind. Just like physical scars, these required constant care. The scar left by brain surgery has always been volatile. Cold, harsh soap, sun, hot water and scratching could all upset it, leaving it raw and painful. After the surgery, I learned to care for this scar, noticing and avoiding those things that harmed it. But I had not realised that I had other, concealed scars that also required care and attention. The wrong conditions could also cause these to flare up and provoke acute pain. The isolation, anxiety and pressure I encountered in Cambridge had exactly this effect, exacerbating existing problems and angering internal scars. I found myself becoming increasingly concerned by my appearance, and the way this would be perceived by others. I was caught up in cycles of worry and dread about future events. I struggled to find self-belief and preserve confidence, and I saw myself as inferior to, and cut off from, fellow students. While I am aware that many undergraduates experience versions of these feelings, they affected me in particularly extreme ways. Throughout much of my second and third years, I found the prospect of leaving my room to take part in social events terrifying. My behaviour became erratic, obsessional and irrational. This was often focused on a strict regime of cleanliness and healthy eating, intended to protect my physical scars and to make me look as healthy as possible. I internalised dietary advice from the internet, feeling panicked if I ate something that could cause me harm. I washed towels again and again to use to dry my scar. Perhaps induced by stress and anxiety, I suffered with bad skin, and my face became red, oily and inflamed, which only added to my self-consciousness. Collectively, these behaviours, feelings and physical symptoms are not difficult to understand considering what I had been through.

Fear and trauma that I had buried were coming to the surface. The internal tumult caused by the shock of finding myself weak and vulnerable was finally revealing itself. But this was not a process that I was in control of. I hadn't learned to tell my new story: to communicate clearly and honestly when I spoke about my illness and its impact. My family and Kate were attentive and caring so they had realised that I was struggling. But I had not found a way to communicate these struggles, as I had not yet named or understood them myself. When I did try to ask for help or to explain my predicament, I found myself almost inarticulate, self-conscious and hesitant as I searched for ways to express myself. The short, simple phrases that I had to resort to, like: 'I'm finding life quite hard', or 'I haven't been feeling myself', felt thin and inadequate. They only gestured to the maelstrom of emotions that was betrayed by my strange behaviour and volatile mood. The suffocating, unsettling awareness of my vulnerability and mortality caused by my illness was not yet something I could translate into language or story.

Despite this, both Kate and my family were steadfast, empathetic companions through the dark moments. I was forced by anxiety and fatigue to narrow my life, limiting the range of people and activities that I was involved with. The kindness and loyalty my family and Kate showed carried me through the remainder of my undergraduate degree. My academic studies also gave me a way to escape troubling thoughts, distracting myself by researching and writing about new, unfamiliar subjects. Increasingly, a strange mismatch developed between my ability to write clearly and insightfully about academic matters, and my capacity to describe the movements of my own heart and soul. My pursuit of greater understanding in the field of academic theology was not leading me towards new ways of interpreting and telling my own story.

Because of this intense focus on my studies, I enjoyed successful results in my exams and assessments. I started to see a career in academia as a natural next step and my plans for the future took shape around this. This imagined future would also include picturing myself married to Kate, who I had become reliant on as a source of kindness and company. We had always shared a loving, trusting bond, so it seemed natural to assume that we would stay together. While marriage and children still seemed distant prospects, they often formed part of my imagined future. But I was soon to be reminded again that my dreams and aspirations were fragile, uncertain things.

In the final year of my studies at Cambridge, my story

took another dramatic turn. Once again, a new chapter began suddenly and unexpectedly. Throughout my time as an undergraduate, my health had remained stable. Whilst the legacies of treatment still affected me, the seizures had stopped, and my condition had stabilised. I had regular MRI scans to monitor my brain and confirm that the tumour had not returned and these continued to find nothing of concern. This cycle of scans provided constant reminders of the fragility of my situation, but I had become accustomed to the nervous waits for results ending in relief. In the springtime holiday before I took my final university exams, I returned home for a brief visit to my family. While I was there, more than four years since the last one, I had a seizure. I had been playing football with my father and brother when I felt the familiar sensation of overwhelming heaviness. Although it had been several years since I had experienced this sensation, I remember realising instantly what was happening. But, as before, there was nothing that I could do to prevent my consciousness from slipping away or gravity from dragging my body onto the grass. Then, I woke up to find myself, yet again, staring up at a paramedic's concerned face, before being rushed to hospital in an ambulance. This visit to the accident and emergency department began with a wait of many hours. Tired, bruised and dirty, with a fierce headache, I sat in a patient bed surrounded by family watching harassed, frantic nurses and doctors rush past. When a doctor eventually arrived to assess me his manner and demeanour made clear that he was working under extreme time pressure. My family and I wanted to describe my medical history in full so that the doctor understood the potential significance of the seizure. But after only a few seconds, and a cursory investigation of my vital signs and blood pressure, the doctor announced that I would be taken for a scan and then left. This brief, unsatisfying encounter did nothing to ease our fears or answer the many questions that were pressing on my mind. Clearly, the seizure indicated that something had changed. In the past, the seizures had been my body's means of warning that the tumour was causing damage and disruption in my brain. I was desperate to know whether this latest seizure meant that the tumour was returning, growing again in harmful, dangerous places. A longer, more sympathetic conversation with a clinician would have given me and my family precious reassurance and clarity in that moment.

The accident and emergency department of a hospital often seems to be the place where the stresses and strains the NHS operates under are most obvious. In my experience, there has never been time or space for calm, attentive care, as healthcare professionals are forced to dash frantically from patient to patient, aware of a building backlog of urgent cases. In this instance, if the doctor had felt he had more time to listen to me, he might have ordered the MRI scan that would have revealed that my tumour was growing again. As it was, I was sent for a different, shorter scan, which did not pick up this concerning change. As soon as I had the scan, the doctor returned and demanded that I vacate my bed and move to a waiting room, as other patients were waiting for beds. I have wondered whether the doctor, seeing a young man who did not look unwell or frail, had decided as soon as he saw me that I was someone to be dealt with and removed as quickly as possible. Usually, it is elderly patients who are given the cruel, inhumane label of 'bed blockers' in NHS hospitals. But I suspect that I was treated in a cursory, impatient manner because I did not appear to be a person in need of urgent treatment: a time-waster occupying a bed that someone else needed more. It is a challenge to look at a 21-year-old man and see someone who may have a life-threatening brain tumour, and I see the doctor's actions as understandable and excusable in deeply difficult circumstances. But I know now that if he had acted differently, it might have changed the course of my life.

After the seizure and my trip to the hospital we were left in a difficult position. It seemed to be very likely that the tumour inside my brain was growing again. An awareness of this left me, my family and Kate with a sense of foreboding, uneasy and frightened as we anticipated bad news. I had one of the routine MRI scans scheduled shortly afterwards and we knew this could confirm our fears. It was as if my life had been placed on hold. I was supposed to be preparing for my final exams, but focusing on anything other than what might be happening in my brain felt impossible. A few days after I had the scan, I received a call from one of the specialist nurses who was supporting me. Usually, I would have a scheduled appointment with a neurologist two weeks after a scan to be told the results, so I knew immediately that something was wrong. The nurse asked me to attend an appointment with the surgeon who had operated on me before. She was not allowed to answer any of my questions as I tried to ascertain why I must see a surgeon. I was left in suspense again, although it was clear that there was cause for concern. I was almost certain that I would require further surgery but until that was confirmed I was left with a feeling of vague, indistinct dread.

It is difficult to prepare to hear disheartening, alarming news unless you are sure that it is coming. So, when I found myself in the surgeon's office again, being told that I would need a third craniotomy, I still felt shaken and shocked. Surgeons tend to be capable of speaking about significant and disturbing things in a calm, professional manner that seems to be at odds with what they're saying. Each time that I have been told I will need surgery I have experienced a bizarre contrast between the steady professionalism of the surgeon and my panicked, frantic interior monologue, as emotional responses and worries swirl in my mind. On this occasion, this contrast became even more pronounced when I heard the surgeon say, in an even, matter-of-fact way: 'and we would like you to be awake'. In my mind this statement was followed by a series of question and exclamation marks, but nothing in the surgeon's tone had suggested it was anything other than a banal, prosaic remark. Only the intent stare he fixed on me betrayed any awareness that proposing awake brain surgery was unusual. He went on to explain that keeping me awake during the procedure would enable them to carry out tests while they were working, helping them to distinguish between tumour and brain. They were eager to remove as much of the tumour as possible and because it was fused to my brain, it was important to guard against accidentally damaging brain cells. As the surgeon described a series of measures to protect me and make me as comfortable as possible during the ordeal, I was still processing the idea of remaining conscious while a team of surgeons opened my skull. I did not hear or absorb much of what was said after I was given this image.

Over the following months, I spent a great deal of time imagining what awake brain surgery might feel like. The surgery had been scheduled after my undergraduate course and exams were finished to allow me to complete my degree. But inevitably, my mind kept returning to the concept of an awake craniotomy. It seemed such an absurd, outrageous idea that I could scarcely believe that it was something I would undergo. I struggled to stop my imagination from probing this strange new prospect. The reactions of friends and family when I told them about the planned surgery only added to my sense of unease. Any mention of brain surgery alone had often been enough to elicit a dramatic reaction, and these were only heightened when I spoke about awake surgery.

This situation meant that the period when my time at Cambridge was ending felt like a hiatus, instead of the final section of a chapter in my life; it had been reframed as a time of waiting, anticipating and worrying. Revision and study provided a welcome distraction again, and my results were better than I had expected. But with the looming threat of the awake craniotomy, this was an ending that felt anticlimactic, without a strong sense of conclusion or achievement. Instead of attending my graduation, I returned home to prepare for the surgery. My fears about the procedure had gradually changed into a desperation to have it done. I knew that it could not possibly be as painful and traumatic as I was picturing, and once I had finally experienced awake surgery, I would be able to give my overactive imagination some respite.

In the end, my suspicions that the surgery would be less awful than I was imagining proved to be well founded. My memories of the six-hour procedure are a surreal blend of pain, exhaustion, conversation and laughter. I had known before it began that there would be an element of human interaction involved to test my brain function, but I had not expected it to take the form of an extended discussion including joking and idle chatter. At the start of the surgery, I was taken into a preparation room to have cannulas, intravenous lines and a urinary catheter inserted into various parts of my body. Throughout the process, an experienced anaesthetist would be present, ready to administer sedatives or to put me to sleep if I became distressed or overwhelmed. This necessitated placing several lines in my veins, ready to deliver drugs. And, as the team warned me before they began, this was a painful and unpleasant process. The practical necessity of inserting a urinary catheter also had to be dealt with while I was awake, which was every bit as embarrassing and uncomfortable as it sounds! It was clear that one member of the team had been instructed to distract me while the others found veins for their needles. This was a thankless task: having to strike up a sufficiently involving, diverting conversation with a stranger. I felt sympathy for him as he fumbled through a list of potential topics: holidays, family, weather, each one faltering then failing as I was distracted by pain. But when I mentioned something that betrayed an interest in football, his eyes lit up. I could see his relief as we found a subject that we could both talk about easily and in depth, and I barely noticed the sharp sting of needles as we exchanged views on our respective teams.

Then, once I was taken into the operating theatre, the surgeon instantly struck up a conversation. Before they could begin cutting away a flap of my skull to gain access to my brain, my head needed to be attached to a harness that would hold it in place. This involved drilling into my skull at three points to fasten it to a metal frame. While they found the right angle for my head and injected local anaesthetic where the frame would be attached, the surgeon asked me about my studies and plans for summer holidays, somehow holding a coherent, jovial conversation while fixing the frame in place. Even as holes were drilled in my skull, we continued to talk like two people getting to know one another over coffee. It became harder to keep up my end of the conversation when they began to use surgical saws to cut into my skull. The anaesthetic numbed the pain, but the sensation and sound would cause my jaw to lock, making it hard to think or speak. As he began the vital part of the procedure, working inside my skull to find the tumour and cut it away, the surgeon described what he was doing in detail, answering my questions and explaining the different stages and processes. A complex array of cameras and monitors allowed the surgeons to work from magnified images of my brain shown on a large screen, making precise incisions. When they reached tissue that could either be brain or tumour, the tests would begin. I would be asked to perform a variety of exercises, such as describing pictures or reciting words, while the tissue was given a small electric shock. Through this, the surgeon could be sure that it was tumour, rather than brain, that was cut away. If my speech failed or my brain function lapsed, they would know that the tissue was brain cells controlling some aspect of my motor skills, speech or cognition.

These tests punctuated the continuing conversation, which had branched out into a range of subjects including hobbies and travel. It is remarkable that the surgeon was able to keep speaking to me in a relaxed, jovial manner while performing such a complex task fraught with risk. A misstep could have triggered a seizure or caused irreparable brain damage, yet he was able to carry out expert, life-saving work while chatting away, only briefly falling silent in difficult moments that required undivided attention. The constant talk helped me to remain calm and distracted for the initial stages of the surgery, and I was able to continue without sedation, so that I remained fully awake and alert. But the pain caused by my neck and head being held fast at an unnatural, uncomfortable angle gradually became hard to bear. I was determined to continue without asking for sedation, however, because I knew that staying fully conscious would make it easier for the tests to be carried out, and that this would enable the surgeon to remove as much tumour as possible.

The purpose behind keeping me awake was to allow the surgeon to cut away tumour safely where it was close to the brain, as any tumour left behind could become cancerous and aggressive. So, I wanted to ensure I did all that I could to make this task as simple as possible. Avoiding sedation became more difficult as time went on, especially once the team started to reattach the skull flap. There are no pain receptors in the brain, so while they worked inside my skull the only source of pain had been the frame and my stiff, aching neck. But the wound required stitches once the flap was in place again. Up to this point, the surgeon had used injections of local anaesthetic to numb the areas of my skin and skull that needed to be cut. But, ironically, these injections themselves caused acute pain. Towards the end of the procedure, with the final stitches still to be sewn into the wound, I felt the effects of the last dose of anaesthetic wearing off. I was offered more but did not want to have another series of painful injections around the tender wound to administer the anaesthetic. This would also have prolonged my time in an increasingly uncomfortable position, dragging out the operation. So, I opted to have the last stitches put in without anaesthetic. In that moment, I was profoundly weary, drained by pain and tension. My powers of endurance were wearing thin. Noticing that I was struggling and close to tears, the anaesthetist, who had been patiently standing by throughout, came to me and took my hand in his. This sudden, unexpected display of tenderness seemed out of keeping with his demeanour.

In consultations before the surgery, he had seemed a quiet, unassuming middle-aged man, reserved and formal in his bedside manner. Yet he showed emotional warmth and acuity in recognising the moment when I was in desperate need of some form of bolstering and reassurance. I was sufficiently surprised and moved by his gesture that it pulled my attention away from the pain caused by the surgeon's needle and thread. This memory is a poignant reminder for me that the NHS is full of caring, attentive individuals, often highly skilled, striving to bring patients comfort and to treat them with generosity and humanity.

By intervening to comfort me when I was at my most vulnerable and desperate, the anaesthetist helped me to reach the end of the surgery without sedation. I was taken to a recovery room and, soon afterwards, my bed was wheeled to a ward where my parents were waiting. They had endured a horrendous wait while I was in surgery, forced for a third time to sit passively as their son went through a complex, potentially life-threatening procedure. Of all the people involved in my surgery, the role that I would least like to have would be that of the anxiously waiting parent. The pain and discomfort that I suffered is surely not comparable to the agony of having to wait as a parent, unable to help or comfort your child while they face such an ordeal, and unsure if you will ever see them alive again.

The relief that I felt once the surgery was complete was profound. I had been lucky again; there were no complications or setbacks in the surgery or my recovery. Once the adrenaline eased, a fatigue that had built over months of exams and anxious anticipation took hold of me. However, I left the hospital with a sense that the problem had been solved. I was due to start a postgraduate course at the University of St Andrews, in Scotland, once the summer was over, and my mind turned to that. I was still not ready to entertain the idea that my story might not unfold smoothly or predictably. I slipped back into the mindset of a young man in the prime of his life, ready to move to a new place and begin the next adventure. Naturally, I chose to dwell on excitement and possibilities rather than potential problems. I was not ready to accept that my life may have become one in which loss and chaos would always be lurking round the next corner. While I began to prepare for my move to Scotland, I received a phone call asking me to attend an appointment with my surgeon. I was not worried by this, as I had expected to be summoned to a post operation debrief. But this did not turn out to be the routine meeting that I had expected.

I arrived ready to be told that the surgery had been a success as I felt well recovered and there had been no signs of any issues during or after the surgery. Yet I detected tension in the room as soon as I entered: a palpable unease. The surgeon and registrar proceeded by telling me that the tests on the tumour sample extracted during surgery had shown that the tumour had changed from grade two to grade three. While it was growing, its threat had intensified, the cells becoming something more dangerous. I later realised that they were – in effect – telling me that I had cancer. But remarkably, the word cancer was not used once during the entire meeting. I remember following the appointment, when I called Kate to tell her the news, she asked whether the change to grade three meant I had cancer and I was unable to answer. I knew that my condition had become more serious, and my prognosis was worse, but I could not say with certainty whether I had cancer. The medical jargon of tumour grades had obfuscated the truth, leaving me confused and hesitant when trying to describe my own condition. Of course, it is important for clinicians to use precise, technical language to diagnose accurately, but this can come at a cost. When this language is not translated for patients, it hinders direct, clear communication. This encounter was just one extreme example of the misunderstandings and confusion that can occur when patients speak to medical experts. What I cannot know is whether this failure of communication had anything to do with an understandable reticence when it came to telling a twenty-one-year-old that they had cancer. If, subconsciously, the surgeon chose to speak about tumour grades rather than cancer, that would be no great surprise. Delivering such news must be deeply difficult and I sympathise with the surgeons and oncologists that have been tasked with telling me heart-breaking things. The fault here lies with the strange, sometimes impenetrable medical lexicon that gives clinicians something to hide behind.

Bizarrely, it was not until I turned up to the hospital that the surgeon had referred me to and realised that it was a cancer centre that I knew for certain I had cancer. This realisation came as a heavy blow. The optimism and excitement I had found having made it through the awake craniotomy was crushed brutally and unexpectedly. I could sense the gravity of the situation and knew that my chances of a normal youth in which I could pursue conventional ambitions and dreams were slipping away. The switch from elated relief to grief and fear was so abrupt that I could not process this development for several weeks. It took time to filter into my consciousness and I remember several occasions after the meeting in which I found myself staring blankly into space, left static and speechless by incomprehension and disorientation. Still feeling dazed,

I attended the meeting with the doctor who was now my assigned oncologist. This meeting brought greater clarity, as the oncologist explained my diagnosis and its implications. I understood that the medical war against my tumour was going to escalate, as a more aggressive tumour called for greater hostility in its treatment. Surgery was just one tool in an oncologist's armoury, to be used first before turning to alternatives. The default in cancer treatment is to match fire with fire, acting swiftly and powerfully to deal with threatening, malignant tumours. A course of radiotherapy was prescribed, followed by a year of chemotherapy. I sat and listened as the next 14 months of my life disappeared, swallowed up by gruelling treatment regimes. I knew that radiotherapy and chemotherapy were notoriously unpleasant forms of treatment with a range of side effects. At this point, the time scale was too much to take in. The idea of spending over a year in treatment was a level of disruption greater than I had yet experienced. The numbness that I had felt since being told my tumour had changed continued, as I struggled to make sense of the drastic changes to my situation and future. I had to try to come to terms with the reality of my cancer, then also to process the loss of my plans to study in Scotland. This amounted to more than I was able to engage with in a single moment, so it took many days until I was able to think or talk about the future in a coherent way. My family and Kate were typically supportive, offering the remarkable form of patient, practical and defiant love that I had come to rely on.

Following my meeting with the oncologist, I had looked up my condition on the reliable websites that she had directed us to as sources of more information on my cancer. Through this research, I discovered that those patients, like me, diagnosed with a grade three astrocytoma had a 50%

chance of being alive in five years, and a 25% chance of being alive in ten years. These statistics were daunting. I felt as if my life had just begun, yet it seemed likely that I had already lived most of the years that I would have. I knew that there were caveats relating to my age and state of health when first diagnosed, but these numbers seemed inescapably clear. When I first came across these statistics, I chose to conceal the pain and fear they provoked. I did not know how to begin speaking to loved ones about my potential death. I was also concerned about the distress it might cause my family and Kate because I assumed that it would provoke the same debilitating despair in them as I felt. For many days, I kept this knowledge to myself, letting it drag me deeper into silent isolation.

Then, one day, I found myself no longer able to conceal this burden. Before my radiotherapy treatment began, my family and I had decided to go on holiday in search of natural beauty to distract and comfort us. While visiting a country house, I became upset and agitated, suddenly overcome with emotion. Noticing this, my mother tried to calm and reassure me by taking me on a walk. She had realised what I had not understood myself: I needed time, space and a private conversation to unburden myself by letting buried feelings come to the surface. After walking for a few minutes on a path beside a canal we sat together on a bench as rain began to fall. With tears in my eyes, I told her about the statistics that I had found and how they had affected me. Predictably, she knew exactly how to respond, hugging me tightly and joining in with my crying. This memory of the first time I spoke to another person about my fear of dying from cancer is still vivid. I recall in sharp detail watching the ripples created by raindrops as they fell into the canal, the smell of the rain on the concrete path, the sensation of being held firmly and lovingly in my mother's arms as I finally released the grief that had accumulated. This was the first moment I had managed to let someone in, bare my soul and show emotional vulnerability. My mother found a way of giving me the opportunity to take that first step towards openness and honesty. She was the first person to hear me try to tell my new story, and I believe that shared moment set me on the path that has led me to the peace and purpose that I have now found.

Chapter 2
BORROWED STORIES

The first time that I tried to tell my new story – to convey how illness had changed my life and sense of self – this was mostly done in the language of tears and hugs. As I sat on that bench next to the canal with my mother, I could only communicate my despondency and loneliness through sobs and my desire for physical closeness. Intuitively, using her maternal instincts and empathy, my mother could interpret this language and respond with the soothing words and reassurance that I required. But there was still a lack of clarity and coherence that frustrated my attempts to unburden myself. I lacked the resources for true storytelling: the words, names, imagery and examples that add substance and depth when we try to tell our story.

The sociologist Arthur Frank describes the problem that I encountered in this first attempt to tell my new story. Frank, a cancer patient himself, wanted to find ways of illuminating the experiences of ill people. He achieved this by drawing attention to the 'need of ill people to tell their stories', as their illness forces them to 'construct new maps and new perceptions of ... the world'.[1] Frank observed that, when we become ill, 'the body sets in motion the need for new stories when its disease disrupts the old stories'.[2] Experiences like vulnerability, pain, dependency or incapacity are, in the first instance, felt physically. But, as Frank noticed, the physical impact of disease reshapes our mental and emotional landscape. As we find our condition affecting who we are and what we do, we look for ways to give voice to these changes. Frank realised that we must avoid becoming alienated from a body that does not match the stories we tell about ourselves.[3] This was the mismatch that I had finally become aware of: the disconnect between the story of an active, healthy, independent young man and the diseased body that frustrated my efforts to hold on to this story. I had to learn how to give my body a voice – to describe the impact of my cancer and its treatment. I could no longer ignore the pain, scarring and weakness that were now part of my everyday existence.

Frank realised that contemporary healthcare institutions like the NHS are not well equipped to help patients find their new story. He saw that 'the modern experience of illness begins when popular experience is overtaken by technical expertise'.[4] He understood, having witnessed this first-hand, that the barrage of medical jargon that patients face when undergoing treatment does not help those left bewildered and shaken by their illness. As patients try to find ways to tell the story of their sickness, obscure technical terms are not what they need. When they encounter new forms of suffering and pain, patients need language that feels relatable, direct and accessible. As I tried to come to terms with my cancer diagnosis, being told about a 'grade 3 anaplastic astrocytoma' did not ease my confusion and disorientation. Even as I began to process the news of my cancer, my oncologist was discussing potential treatments, introducing me to radiotherapy and chemotherapy. Details of these were also conveyed in language that was unfamiliar and opaque to me, so that I struggled to make sense of what was happening and where my life was now leading.

An alternative means of understanding my struggles at this point is offered by Austrian psychiatrist Viktor Frankl. Frankl argued that a patient's 'will to meaning' should always be treated as a 'primary concern' when trying to protect their mental health. He believed that the 'search for meaning' was an essential part of every person's life and identity. He recognised that serious illness could disrupt and prevent this search, and that this could lead to mental health problems including depression.[5] Frankl's theories on the search for meaning are a useful way of understanding the existential impact of a disease like cancer. Because I could not find a sense of 'meaning' in what was happening to me, because I did not feel purpose, certainty, hope or acceptance, I was not able to speak about my experiences with confidence or optimism.

Unfortunately, Frankl succumbs to a familiar form of pessimism when he writes about how we might help ill people search for meaning. He declares that we are now living in an 'existential vacuum' because of the loss of the 'traditions and values' that religion once supplied.[6] This sweeping dismissal of contemporary society and culture is indicative of his belief that the modern era is one of 'meaninglessness, depersonalisation and dehumanisation'.[7] In Frankl's view, there is not much 'out there' to support or enrich a patient's search for meaning, as we have lost sight of the sources of meaning that we used to turn to. He does not seem willing to entertain the possibility that alternative sources of meaning might be emerging in new places, or that some of the traditions and values he believes are lost could have been preserved, reimagined and passed on through new mediums.

Arthur Frank, however, offers a more hopeful

perspective. His focus on storytelling allows him to recognise potential sources of meaning and inspiration beyond traditional ones like organised religion. Spending time with other ill people, Frank noticed that when patients lack the 'narrative resources' to express what they have experienced, they 'borrow' stories.[8] When aspects of their experiences fall outside the boundaries of what they can easily communicate, ill people need help. Hearing other stories that might provide the resources required to describe their own experiences is usually how these patients begin to find their voice and tell a new story that accurately conveys what they are thinking and feeling. Having found 'flexible' stories that can be reshaped to fit their personal experiences, ill people tell new stories that are complex composites. They 'remix borrowed fragments' from other stories that they have heard, creating their own unique illness narrative.[9] As Frank watched this process of 'perpetual reinvention' take place, he realised that 'every story borrows from other stories'.[10] We all require external sources of inspiration to be able to tell our story. Family, friends and fellow patients are all potential suppliers of the borrowed 'fragments' that patients need to piece together a new story when illness disrupts their old life story and leaves them searching for meaning. And what Frank recognised is that it is not just past traditions and values that can help an ill person to rediscover meaning and purpose.

Yet Frank also identified another important source of the kind of flexible stories that can be borrowed from by ill people struggling to tell their story. He shows an awareness of the influence of mass media products such as film and television in contemporary society, observing that when we search for inspiration today, 'most people's poets are the creators of mass media stories'.[11] Our 'poets' – the people we turn to when we need help interpreting or describing our experiences – are often those who create television series, popular films or bestselling novels. Whether consciously or subconsciously, we find fragments in the stories we watch or read that apply to our own lives, then incorporate them in our storytelling. Frank also draws attention to the value of these kind of shared, popular stories when they provide a 'common space' in which people can relate to each other.[12] As an aid for communication and connection, stories that touch on aspects of our personal experiences can provide a starting point for important conversations by making self-expression easier. Serious illness often adds new barriers and complications to our relationships, and borrowing from 'flexible' stories can play a key role by aiding mutual understanding.

This discussion of borrowed stories and modern mass media paints a very different picture to Frankl's gloomy warnings about our era of meaninglessness and loss of the traditions and values that helped us to navigate illness and death. Frank's work highlights the different resources available to ill people in contemporary society, explaining how our communities and culture can help us to find a new story to tell about death and disease. There is a stronger sense in Frank's work of the ingenuity and imagination that ill people often show when it comes to finding a sense of self and purpose amid the chaos caused by their diagnosis. Frank is also refreshingly optimistic about the capacity for mass media stories – the things most people watch, read or listen to – to help in the search for a new 'destination and map'. By paying close attention to patients and listening to them, he started to see how meaning-making can happen through everyday encounters with friends, family and fellow patients, or even the right book, novel or television series.

BORROWED STORIES

My personal story is a good example of how this can happen in practice. After my cancer diagnosis, I gradually discovered that the inspiration and resources I needed to begin constructing a new life story were all around me. Without searching proactively for stories to borrow from, I came across people and narratives that enabled me to begin telling my own story. Often unexpectedly, I discovered stories that helped me to express the impact of cancer on my body, mind and soul. In the hope that it might prove valuable for another ill person searching for a story, I am going to use this chapter to describe how I found my story, offering this as something for others to borrow from. Explaining how I stumbled upon fragments in other stories as I pieced together my new story might give an ill person the impetus to begin their own search, looking for the materials that will enable them to process and express their experiences. Tracing my development towards clarity, coherence and confidence as a storyteller will add detail to the message of hope that I am trying to convey and help to explain what Frank meant by 'borrowed stories'.

I first started to find fragments of a new story in the period after my cancer diagnosis in which I endured 7 weeks of radiotherapy, followed by a year of chemotherapy. These treatments were unpleasant and arduous, but they did provide me with something crucial when it came to reconstructing my story: time. The radiotherapy necessitated daily visits to the hospital for treatment sessions but within this schedule there were gaps for rest and recovery, as well as vigils in hospital waiting rooms that frequently stretched for several hours. The chemotherapy was organised into 12 4-week cycles. Each cycle began with 5 days of taking the chemotherapy drugs, then this was followed by 23 days of recovery. The cumulative effects of the radiation fired at my brain and the toxicity of the chemotherapy drugs meant that I was feeling lethargic and listless for much of this 14-month period. The collateral damage caused by the treatments forced my body into a state of permanent healing that left little room for excitement or exertion. This meant that I had many stretches of time to fill with peaceful, undemanding activity in which I felt unable to do anything more ambitious than thinking, reading, watching television or talking to my family. Yet what I would eventually discover is that when it came to finding meaning in my experiences of illness, and learning to tell my new story, each of these activities would prove vital. While my body recovered from physical trauma, my explorations in novels and television drama, as well as my discussions with loved ones, contributed to a process of spiritual and emotional healing.

In his enticingly-titled book, *The End of Your Life Book Club*, Will Schwalbe describes how, while his mother was dying of cancer, reading books gave them a 'way into' difficult conversations about sensitive subjects like death and grief.[13] Schwalbe uses the story of his time with his dying mother as an illustration of the power of stories we read to initiate, and then enrich, important processes of self-examination and communication, especially for people affected by serious illness. He relates how borrowed fragments from a wide variety of novels, memoirs and non-fiction books gave him a way of engaging with his mother's terminal condition in a meaningful and empathetic way. As Schwalbe's mother died, these fragments helped her to tell her life story, including the final chapter as cancer brought it to an end. Books provided the 'common space' that Frank refers to when he writes about borrowed stories: the starting point for the painful conversations that they had to have.

Despite being an author and editor, Schwalbe

acknowledges that television is becoming an increasingly prominent part of our emotional and spiritual lives.[14] And I found many television series resonating with my personal experiences of cancer. Faced with a year of chemotherapy and convalescence, I found myself with time to watch *Breaking Bad*, the latest Netflix mega-hit. By chance, I had chosen to watch a long, detailed series about a man's reaction to a terminal cancer diagnosis. While I had picked up a few plot details from friends, I did not realise until I watched the first episode that *Breaking Bad* is a story all about the existential, emotional impact of cancer. Walter White (played by Bryan Cranston) is a quiet, unassuming chemistry teacher who suddenly discovers that he is dying of incurable lung cancer. Driven by panic and denial, he decides to conceal his diagnosis from his family, opting instead to use his chemical expertise to begin manufacturing high quality methamphetamine in a reckless attempt to raise money to fund his healthcare and secure his family's future. As I spent many hours watching Walter become trapped in self-imposed isolation, slipping gradually into criminality and immorality, I began to see my own inclination towards silence and self-reliance in a new light. In the story of Walter's lonely descent, motivated by desperation and a stubborn belief in his capacity to fight cancer alone, I could recognise the dangers of turning inwards and refusing to seek support from family. The confusion and distress Walter's deception causes also alerted me to the ways that my insularity could affect loved ones, creating an unfamiliar sense of distance and detachment. Reading different examples of cancer patients' testimonies, the contrast between the 'World of Cancer' and everyday, easy family life is often emphasised.[15] Being a cancer patient can feel lonely and isolating. Yet in *Breaking Bad*, Walter White makes no attempt to bridge the gap between the World of Cancer and his family life, even creating new boundaries and intentionally cutting himself off from his wife and son.

As I watched this, wrapped up in over 60 hours of television drama, questions began to form in my mind. What if I was making the same mistakes as Walter? Could I act differently and make alternative choices? How else could someone respond to incurable cancer? Whilst I was borrowing from Walter's story, using his behaviour and language to name my own fear and denial, I could also see how these fragments might form part of a more hopeful, constructive narrative. *Breaking Bad* had given me a framework for my new story, as well as a starting point. But it was also challenging me. Where Walter found only despair and nihilistic recklessness, I could see opportunities for allowing the love and generosity of others to change life with cancer. And this was leading me to reflect on my story. In particular, the moments when Walter deliberately deceives his son, Walter Jr., were setting in motion important thought processes. Walter Jr. ('Junior' to his family, and later Flynn), played by RJ Mitte, is a courageous young man struggling with physical limitations caused by cerebral palsy. He is the moral and emotional core of a family life based on mutual dependence. As Junior sees his father's deceptions start to undermine the trusting, open relationship he cherishes, he advocates passionately for a return to unequivocal honesty. As he grapples with health problems and bodily dysfunction, Junior clearly values vulnerability in others, wanting his father to accept and acknowledge his own suffering and struggles, and consequent need for support. After learning about his father's cancer diagnosis, Junior notices that Walt is trying to take on the emotional and physical burden of his disease alone, rejecting the love and care his family and friends would willingly provide. Junior has learned to cherish mutual dependence, but his father has not.

Occasionally, the viewer is given a glimpse of what could happen if Walt also learned to embrace his need for support. In a rare moment of vulnerability, Walt suddenly tells his son about his own experience of seeing his father in hospital dying of Huntington's disease. The unexpected, poignant qualities of this image of a weeping, battered cancer patient highlight what Walt has been missing up to this point: the shared understanding which submitting to weakness and reliance makes possible. When Walt tries to reinstate the façade of the strong, solitary cancer-warrior the next day, his son's reaction serves to reinforce this message: 'at least last night you were real' (Season 4, Episode 10: 'Salud'). Walt treats his acknowledgement of anxiety as an aberrant display of vulnerability. Yet Walter Jr. suddenly sees his father's real, true self open to meaningful connection, before it is obscured again. The audience is reminded that they are seeing symbols of what could have been: fragments of the loving relationships Walt could have depended on.

Junior's perspective on what is 'real' while living with disease and disability became a fragment that I borrowed as I began to piece together my new story. His words felt especially resonant because of their relevance to my own family life. My younger brother, Alfie, had always occupied a similar role to Junior in our family: an anchoring and uplifting figure whose courage rooted us in love and shared hope. After Alfie was born 16 weeks prematurely, he survived a long stay in a high-dependency unit, as well as a life-threatening brain haemorrhage, and has become a sociable, capable and admirable young man.

As he has grown from a tiny new-born weighing less than a kilogram into an athletic, 6-foot-tall man, Alfie has become a binding force at the heart of our tight-knit family unit. With a unique blend of honesty and humour, Alfie has shown how dependence on others can breed strength, as he has allowed us to share in the challenges caused by his complex, acquired learning difficulties and physical impairment.

Noting the parallels between Junior and Alfie, I could recognise how I was – like Walt – losing sight of the shared vulnerability that Alfie had helped us to cultivate. By resorting to denial and silence I was not staying true to the family ethic that had grown out of Alfie's attitude to adversity. As Walter's poor decisions reminded me of the choices that I had made, I realised that I could not survive or flourish without inviting my family into my World of Cancer. I decided to take a different path from Walter. Tentatively, I tested out new levels of openness, admitting to thoughts and feelings that I had previously buried. The boundaries that I had set up around my innermost being became more permeable. And as this happened, I found myself rediscovering new forms of relationship that felt more 'real'.

As this first fragment of my new story fitted into place, these reflections led to a deeper level of exploration. By bringing myself closer to the support, loving care and guidance that my family offered, I exposed myself to different perspectives on my condition. Before my health problems, conversations with my parents had been a reliable way for me to process and respond to challenges of all kinds. As sounding boards and conversation partners, they were patient, sympathetic and insightful – ever-ready to offer counsel or consolation. And when it came to working out what I wanted my life story to become, they were invaluable sources of wisdom and experience. As a journalist and radio producer and presenter, my father, Chris, understood the importance of telling and hearing stories. My initial attempts to find meaning in my experiences of cancer were supported and enriched by this expertise. His appreciation of stories as a complex, rich composite of imagery, dialogue and emotion enabled him to guide me towards a new narrative. He helped me to draw out the key themes and moments that I could build my storytelling around with tact, understanding and a journalist's eye for the key details. My first course of radiotherapy required me to walk up the hill between my family home and the hospital so that I could have radiation treatment every day. Often, my father kindly accompanied me on these trips to the hospital, and this gave us opportunities to share stories and begin to think through my illness and its implications.

One of the topics that we returned to frequently while walking and talking was the defiance Alfie had shown in overcoming a profoundly difficult start to his life. I clearly remember one such conversation with my father that eventually led to the idea of the 'inner baby'. As we reflected on the nature of modern healthcare, my father told me about his memories of a night when the tiny, fragile, new-born Alfie had nearly died. Having reached the point at which she felt she could not do anything more for Alfie, the doctor had told my parents that Alfie's survival was dependent on his 'inner baby'. In other words, Alfie's condition had reached the point at which the powers of medical science end, and the potency of an individual's will to survive becomes the vital factor. Alfie's deep, exuberant life force became the sustaining medicine that kept him alive that night. This short story revealed much about the limits of evidence-based medicine, as well as the capacities of the human spirit. Alfie, in his weakness and vulnerability, showed that our souls can allow us to hold on to life when drugs and treatments prove ineffective. He gave us a glimpse into the spiritual, mysterious realm that medical science cannot access. And he also demonstrated that a patient in hospital can be an active, decisive participant in their own care and survival; through sheer force of will, and a refusal to allow his inchoate existence to end before it was even supposed to start, Alfie kept himself alive. Talking about Alfie's remarkable story with my father helped me to see how it was relevant to my situation. Whilst – from a clinical perspective – my prognosis was bleak, Alfie's story showed how we can find hope from beyond the science and statistics. The infectious *joie de vivre* that continues to characterise Alfie's life is a constant reminder of the inner baby that chose to embrace life in defiance of poor odds. I saw that if I borrowed the idea of the inner baby, searching for defiant hopefulness in the core of my being, I might also live a life ungoverned by the doom-laden pronouncements about my chances of a long life and enduring health. Inspired by Alfie, I realised that I could make choices, and that living with disease and disability can be done in many ways.

It was not only Alfie's story that led me towards this shift in perspective. My mother, Jane, was also a remarkable example of a person who had refused to be daunted or diminished by health problems. Talking to her about my life with cancer, I learned more about how she had chosen to live a full, active life, despite the terrible traffic accident that left her with two badly broken legs. Her response to being struck and seriously injured by a van when only six years old had been to pursue sports competition and physical challenges with relish and courage: hockey, swimming, cycling, hiking. Although the accident had left her with one leg significantly shorter than the other, her prowess as a hockey player was such that she competed in the men's league at university. Such feats are typical of a life story that has come to be defined by persistence, strength, resolve and bravery – by a spirited inner baby that never hesitated when facing new challenges. A more recent development in this story that proved particularly revealing and inspiring for me was the pioneering surgery that my mother underwent to correct the disparity in length between her legs. The Ilizarov technique involves breaking the shorter leg, then using a metal frame gradually to increase the leg's length as the bones heal. This necessitates a painful, prolonged period after surgery during which the patient is responsible for adjusting the frame to stretch their own leg. As a young boy, watching my mother face this ordeal was an important formative experience; her steady resilience as she struggled with a painful, life-limiting routine gave me an example of how it is possible to take suffering in your stride, finding a healthy balance between emotional openness and quiet endurance. She refused to allow anger, pain or frustration to define her life during that period of recovery and transformation. Like Alfie, she showed how spirited determination can enable a patient to shape the course of their treatment, drawing on inner resources more powerful than anything that doctors can prescribe.

At one stage during the treatment process, my mother was told by a physiotherapist that, because of the physical trauma caused by the Ilizarov procedure, she was unlikely ever to be able to walk again without the aid of a crutch. When this happened, I can recall, vividly, the shock and distress this caused. For someone with the energy and vivaciousness of Jane this was an awful prospect. Yet this was a prognosis that she chose not to accept. It became the pivotal point at which she took hold of her situation as her inner baby stirred. My memory of her face after the physiotherapy appointment, bleached with shock and concern, has since become a moment that I can recognise as a starting point. Just as Alfie chose, when clinicians could no longer help him to live and thrive, Jane decided that she would walk, swim, cycle, hike, and even run again. Today, she is fiercely, remarkably healthy and active. Her physical capability stands as a testament to the spiritual depths that she called on when faced with a bleak prognosis.

As I talked about these two stories with my father, walking back and forth from the radiotherapy sessions, something important happened. I noticed the two narratives drawing together, coalescing around ideas that felt relevant and significant. With my father's help, I was discerning something that I could borrow from as I tried to respond to my own situation. The themes of brave, soulful autonomy and intentionality that emerged in both stories gave me a means of beginning to understand and describe my desire to regain control of the course of my life: to become author of my story again. I wanted to be something more than the passive recipient of a doctor's prognosis, and I was realising that two of my family members had shown how that can be achieved. Separately and uniquely, each offered a model for an alternative way to respond to disease and disability.

But it was only through the process of reflective storytelling initiated and guided by my dad that I reached this realisation. Before I could step out of the insularity and fearful silence that had characterised my reaction to cancer, I had to hear and reflect on other people's stories. These people were close to home but could still provide the impetus and inspiration to drive my change from passive patient to active, inquisitive storyteller. Without their influence, I may never have reached the point where I felt

I could take control of my story, learning to talk openly, clearly and meaningfully about my experiences of cancer. Finding this inspiration in their stories also encouraged me to begin searching further afield. What if there were sources of stories beyond my family and *Breaking Bad*? I began to wonder if there might be an endless, interwoven tapestry of stories 'out there' that might help me to find my voice and understand my experiences. I started actively seeking out stories about cancer, fictional and real, finding these in novels, films, memoirs, autobiographies, newspapers. This also led me to recognise that, when I was diagnosed with cancer, I had become part of a community. Few lives are untouched by cancer, and my inclination towards privacy and introversion had prevented me from noticing that my disease gave me a strange bond with many other people – people who I could learn and borrow from.

As I explored these exciting new connections, one friendship in particular gave me a clear sense of the beauty and affirmation that can emerge from the bonds that cancer creates. My Aunt Rachel, a literature professor, was supervising a young Italian woman who happened to be interested in the same questions about fictional stories and cancer that were running through my mind. Through painful personal experiences, Vale had become aware of the ways in which fictional stories can help us to find meaning in our own experiences of cancer. Insightfully and kindly, Rachel put Vale and me in contact, giving us an opportunity to discuss this shared interest. As soon as we began to exchange emails, I knew that I had found a kindred spirit. Not only that, but I had also been put in contact with another young person affected by cancer, a person who had met tragedy and suffering with perceptiveness, courage and imagination. In emails that were almost poetic, Vale explained to me how literature had been like a 'lighthouse' for her during her experiences of cancer, offering stories that illuminated dark, difficult moments while helping her to find a path through painful times. This lighthouse metaphor is one that I have borrowed many times as I have sought to understand and convey the importance of fiction as a resource for my own storytelling.

As our bond and mutual understanding grew, Vale also told me about a project in which she had used a guided tour of an art gallery to help a group of women to process and speak about their experiences of breast cancer. As I was beginning to see how a wide range of stories and artworks could offer important resources to ill people left confused and silent by their condition, Vale gave me clear, thought-provoking examples of how this can happen. The stories she shared refined and expanded my own ideas; there was much in her vision and imaginative energy for me to borrow from as I explored new territory. Vale had shown how someone affected by cancer can help others to find their own stories, passing on insights acquired through experience. Drawing on the lighthouse of literature for guidance, Vale found a path towards meaning that she could lead others along.

I was lucky to be one of the people who could follow this path, and, with Vale's encouragement, I found myself drawn into the world of cancer stories. Wrapped up in the diversity and detail of individual stories – real or imagined – I came across a wealth of different sources of hope, meaning and consolation. This became nourishment and incitement for my soul – my inner baby – as I found my storytelling voice.

After coming through a daunting 14 months of radiotherapy and chemotherapy, I had decided to resume my academic career at the University of St Andrews as a member of the excitingly named Institute for Theology, Imagination and the Arts (ITIA). My interest in theology had developed into a desire to study how literary fiction can enrich our spiritual searching. The skill and insight with which authors like Dostoevsky, George Eliot and Primo Levi used their talents to shed light on our spiritual, existential struggles had arrested my attention. Their vivid, thrilling renderings of guilt, doubt, ambiguity, loneliness and faith became the subject that captured my scholarly imagination. It is surprising and embarrassing that it took me almost a year of studying before I noticed that my academic interests and personal illness story were converging around a common theme. Whilst my time as a postgraduate student was devoted to trying to understand how stories by remarkable authors could reveal the complexities of our innermost thoughts and feelings, my journey as a cancer patient was being determined by the impact of such stories on my life. Stories and storytelling had become the focus of both my intellectual and spiritual explorations. But there was an important difference between these two forms of exploration. Whilst my academic study of stories was limited by set texts, recommended readings and convention, my personal searching could lead in all directions. Academic courses inevitably focused on 'classics' and notionally 'high' art, but real-life exploration is not constrained by predetermined categories and prejudices. I had found that I was just as likely to come across a story that helped me to understand myself and my illness scrolling through Netflix as I was browsing Penguin Classics. I had found so many different types of storytelling in a wide range of places. As I considered the possibility of bringing together my academic and personal exploration of stories in a formal, intentional way, I wanted to ensure this would not limit the scope of my search. As I sought out stories that could help me and others to find meaning while living with cancer, I wanted to be able to look everywhere.

Fortunately, I was already a member of an academic institute characterised by the kind of generous openmindedness that is receptive to new ideas, enabling students to undertake novel, unconventional research projects. In fact, the teaching at ITIA often actively encouraged me to step outside the boundaries of academic convention. I could sense that I was in a space that could support the kind of search for stories that I wanted to begin. So, I applied to a PhD programme, proposing to research how the arts could be used in the spiritual care of cancer patients. I used vague, open terms like 'the arts' and 'spiritual care' to ensure that this project could take into account a diverse range of stories and experiences. I was using words and ideas that were open to interpretation, and mean different things to different people, but that was the point. I wanted to design a project that could accommodate the fascinating subjectivity and unpredictability of each cancer patient's unique story, as well as the full range of stories that ill people borrow from. I hoped that this would allow me to be open to unforeseen discoveries and unexpected developments as my theories were tested against the messiness and complexity of human life and illness.

Looking for people to test my ideas on brought me into contact with Maggie's cancer care centre in Dundee. As I tried to find other cancer patients who might be interested in my research into stories, I realised that Maggie's centres, devoted to the holistic care and support of cancer patients, were an obvious place to look. People come to Maggie's seeking community and conversation; the centres are designed to create opportunities for connection and reflection that hospital buildings do not afford. The idea of Maggie's centres was first conceived by Maggie and Charles Jencks, two artists, while Maggie was dying of cancer. They believed that cancer patients should have a place to go that offered calm, beauty, peace, and emotional and practical support. Often designed by talented architects, Maggie's centres are intended as both a contrast and complement to hospital cancer wards, giving patients respite from the clinical environment and a different form of care more focused on a person's emotional and psychological needs. Because Maggie's brings people together in groups, giving patients a safe, comforting environment in which to meet, they are places in which stories can be exchanged. As soon as I began to visit the Maggie's centre in Dundee, I realised that this was a place where I could be heard and understood, as well as hear other stories that would help me to tell my own. I joined a support group for men affected by cancer, travelling to Dundee every Monday to hear tales of loss, suffering, anger and grief. For the first time, I heard other men naming and describing some of the powerful, painful feelings that I had buried for so long. I was deeply affected by the generosity and sympathy shown by the other members of the group, most of whom were several decades older than me. The courage and candour they showed when telling their own stories, and the attention and compassion they offered listening to me, became vital to my own storytelling.

This group environment of honesty and support, vulnerability and humanity, was the first place that I tried to harness the power of stories. I wanted to see if I could enhance the process of storytelling that was already happening. I began to introduce the members of the men's group to a range of different stories about cancer, each using a different medium and style: television dramas, novels, sitcoms, Hollywood films. Whilst I was worried that these fictional, 'fake' stories might be regarded as unwelcome intrusions, they proved popular and sparked conversation, self-reflection and lively debate. Naturally and instinctively, the men borrowed from these fictional explorations of life with cancer to talk about their own experiences, drawing comparisons with characters and storylines, or adopting language and imagery from the television series and films we watched together. At times, it even seemed like the fictional stories were making room for topics to be raised that might otherwise have remained untouched. I found that I could deliberately choose stories that would lead us towards specific subjects that were sensitive and needed approaching delicately. When the fictional stories about cancer became part of the conversations, something was being added; new ideas and perspectives were coming into our discussions. There was a freshness and energy to the meetings when I brought different stories in from outside – storytelling flowed faster, charged with meaning and purpose. The stories these men told were already profound, important and inspiring, but they took on new depth and detail when interwoven with a new collection of imaginative resources to borrow from. I had discovered that my belief in the power of stories was well founded.

Having learned that fictional stories could enhance the storytelling that took place in Maggie's centres, I wanted to test this further. Drawing on my conversations with Maggie's staff, I began to design a new resource: *The Maggie's Fiction Library*. The 'fiction library' resource was intended to give anyone who came into a Maggie's centre the opportunity to use fictional stories to explore their own experiences of cancer. It provided stories to borrow from (novels and DVDs of television series and films), and an accompanying guidebook suggesting how these stories could help someone to try to understand and speak about the ways cancer had affected them. The guidebook connected questions and themes to specific stories, showing how an imagined fictional story can shed new light on areas of experience that are important for many cancer patients. I wanted to use the guide to pass on what I had learned, helping others to find the stories that could become a 'lighthouse' for them as they struggled through darkness. As I created then enacted this scheme, it was frustrating to have to operate within the confines of academic practice. I had no choice but to use the forms, frameworks and guidelines set out by the university to ensure that researchers behaved in an ethical, appropriate manner when working with other people. I appreciated the importance of acting with care and caution when dealing with sensitive matters, asking cancer patients to explore personal and traumatic experiences, but the one-size-fits-all approach that I had to follow felt unsatisfactory. The dull, flat bureaucracy of tick-box forms jarred with the generosity and honesty that I encountered as people shared their stories. When they described their responses to the fictional cancer storylines, those involved in the trial were expansive, insightful and candid in ways the formulaic questionnaires could not always contain.

For instance, one participant in the trial told me how coming across a character in a television series who reflected their own fear, loneliness and denial after diagnosis led them to seek a closer relationship with their family. Another participant spoke about novels that helped them to understand the 'rollercoaster' of life with cancer and the moments of joy they found amongst pain and chaos. Maggie's staff involved in the trial described finding new ideas for providing patients with counselling and psychological healing in the fictional stories. This feedback, anonymised to protect the people who told me highly personal information, gave me a powerful sense of hope and purpose. Hearing about these meaningful, important interactions between fictional cancer stories and the real stories of people affected by cancer galvanised my research, presenting me with voices that encouraged and deepened my investigations. Once more, I found myself borrowing from other people, hearing them express ideas I had been struggling to pin down or express myself. In later chapters, I plan to weave the voices of participants in the fiction library trial into my explorations of key themes in my own cancer story. In doing so, I hope to make clear how much I am indebted to the words and ideas of others for the meaning that I have found while living with, and dying of, cancer.

Yet this also became the beginning of a new chapter in my story as, for the first time, I realised that I had something to offer to others. The discoveries that I had made while searching for stories about cancer could – it appeared – be valuable and revealing for other patients. I understood that, through stories, I could offer others living with cancer forms of insight, consolation and meaning that they could borrow from to tell their own story.

The start of this new chapter happened to coincide with the beginning of the COVID pandemic and this health crisis was to become a period in which I learned a great deal more about cancer, storytelling, and the new direction that my life was taking. When the first UK lockdown was announced, I had been preparing for a research internship in which I would move back for a time to live with my parents and brother, who had moved to the North East of England. I would spend time with a small Northumberland-based cancer support group (the NCSG) trying to use my research and ideas to add to the programme of therapy, meetings and activities the group offered to members. My work with Maggie's had given me a desire for more of the human interaction that was bringing my ideas to life, challenging me and enlightening me. So, I had arranged to spend several months with the support group for people affected by cancer, learning from their stories and from their responses to my ideas. But, following an initial period of in-person meetings, the sudden announcement of an unprecedented national lockdown forced us into separation.

After overcoming the initial shock this caused, I began to realise that all my plans for the internship would need to be rethought. These were based around gathering, storytelling and socialising in person. At first, this seemed like an insurmountable obstacle. I could not see any way to make possible the kind of interactions that I had been aiming to encourage. But once the mass switch to online virtual forms of meeting began to gather pace, I started to recognise this as an opportunity. What if I could use technology to create spaces in which people affected by cancer could support one another by telling, hearing and discussing stories? It seemed inevitable that something would be lost in the shift to virtual interaction, but might this also make new things possible? For cancer patients, meeting in person has always been complicated. Travel is often fraught with difficulty, and concerns about compromised immune systems and the risks of viral infection were already familiar for cancer patients before COVID arrived. This means that the pleasures of sharing a space with other people can come at a cost and I realised that I had a chance to test out alternative options.

As I discussed the problem of lockdown with the support group committee, an idea began to take shape: a virtual space that used stories to create conversation and maintain connection between group members. The committee contained several people who had been professional caregivers and therapists, and their experience and expertise helped me to see how I might put my research into practice in this situation. Once more, I was borrowing, drawing on the insight, memory and knowledge of other people. With their guidance, I designed a group on a social media platform that would use fictional stories to encourage members to explore and share their experiences of cancer and also of life in lockdown. By using imagined stories to introduce sensitive subjects, I hoped I could give the impression of a space in which personal, emotional matters could be talked about.

I soon found myself taking part in lively, frank online discussions on themes like loneliness, grief, time and mortality. Each week, I would choose a novel, film or television series for the group to read or watch, then draw out particular themes or questions from the story for the group to reflect on. As we all struggled to reconcile ourselves to distance and separation, this became something to do and to think about. It also seemed to give members of the group the freedom and confidence to disclose feelings and unburden themselves. As the fictional stories touched on subjects that resonated with their experiences, it appeared to give the members the permission to speak that they had desired. Remarkable levels of trust and intimacy quickly developed in this online setting as the storytelling gathered pace, flowing naturally out of discussions of fictional narratives and characters. I was surprised to discover this intensity of bond could be mediated through a virtual platform, but the power of stories could clearly work in this form of space, too.

Several of the people in the virtual group were strangers to me, whom I had not met in person, but after interacting with them through this unusual, improvised gathering, I felt that they had become close friends and confidants. As many of the group expressed with clarity and eloquence, the flow of stories eased the pain of isolation and met, to some extent, our natural need for community and companionship. At times, the textual, disembodied nature of our interactions felt frustratingly limited – stripped of the immediacy of physical proximity and the nuance of tone and body language – but our encounters still felt meaningful. There was a therapeutic, cathartic aspect of the group that emerged out of the exchange of stories, as trauma and tragedy were disclosed, acknowledged and affirmed. Especially during a time in which we all felt unsettled and frightened by the pandemic, this continuing sense of support and community felt vital. For many of the group, the constant reminders of death and disease that COVID provided brought memories of suffering and grief to the surface. Collaboratively, we learned how support could be offered through a virtual medium, discovering how to convey compassion and companionship when typed text was all that was available. Woven into these exchanges was always language and imagery from the novels, series and films that I introduced to the group. To protect the privacy of the group members, I cannot disclose specific examples of the rich storytelling that took place in this digital space. But challenging and unprecedented circumstances forced us to find new ways of forging connections, and we were surprised by how spiritually, emotionally satisfying these screen-based encounters proved to be.

My experiences of running and participating in the online group served to intensify my interest in storytelling. This also alerted me to how tightly intertwined my personal search for meaning and my academic explorations had become. As I took part in the group, I was growing and learning in a cerebral, intellectual sense, but I was also gaining self-knowledge and growing in emotional and spiritual maturity. The people that I interacted with through my keyboard were teaching me about myself and the world. I believe the academic ideal of a 'rational', detached researcher observing in an impartial manner is deceptive and detrimental. In my admittedly limited experience, there is always a personal dimension to our research, and the best research often happens when the researcher is openly invested in, and passionate about, their subject. The situations that my academic work was drawing me into, as well as the people it was bringing me into contact with, were contributing to my development as a person. As my academic career and private life converged, it gave my story a clarity and sense of direction that had been missing for many years. So, it seemed natural to treat these as two strands of my existence that were uniting in a single search.

This search led me to seek out new ways of encouraging storytelling amongst cancer patients. I felt called to act on the discoveries that I had made about the power of fictional stories. Still constrained by lockdowns, I decided to continue trying to create virtual spaces in which stories could be exchanged. I felt energised by the success of my work with the local cancer support group during the first lockdown and this made me determined to treat social distancing as a challenge rather than a problem. I was also aware that if the academic world was going to take my work seriously, I needed evidence. While it does not seem right to attach words like 'evidence' or 'data' to the forms of heartfelt, honest storytelling that I witnessed, academic disciplines investigating different forms of care still use this kind of language and demand empirical, verifiable 'proof' of the validity of new approaches to patient care. So even though I was intentionally placing distance between my research and the demands of evidence-based medicine, I still had to conform to this requirement for 'data'.

In this instance data meant evidence collected in formalised, pre-approved ways: the same forms and frameworks that I had to employ for the fiction library trial. I could not use the voices of NCSG members from the virtual reading group because that had been an improvised creation, fluid and flexible by necessity as we responded to new challenges. Instead, I devised a plan to use 'focus groups' to record voices testifying to the power of fictional cancer storylines to enrich storytelling and create connection. With the help of Maggie's staff and the NCSG committee, I arranged to meet cancer patients and test out my ideas on them in virtual groups. Because I set these meetings up as formal trials, securing consent from all involved to record the meeting, this would produce evidence that I could use in my research and in publications. The bureaucracy this entailed, as well as the virtual medium, made it hard to make these meetings seem natural and comfortable. I often found myself working with groups of six or seven assembled strangers, which made encouraging storytelling and honesty a daunting task. Yet I soon learned that these barriers to easy communication could be overcome by the right fictional story. While the atmosphere at the virtual meetings was usually tense and hesitant at first, as I struggled to contain my nerves and the participants tried to understand what they were being asked to do, the mood transformed once I introduced an excerpt or example from a story that resonated with the experiences of those present. Comments, anecdotes and memories would instantly begin flowing as the participants warmed to a new theme. Powerful, passionate storytelling would begin, with any sense of inhibition set aside.

In these moments, I felt that I was witnessing something remarkable, almost sacred. The strength and depth of connection that surged across the virtual space was humbling to witness. In one focus group, I remember beginning with the impression that I was boring and confusing the six women present on the Zoom call – none of whom I had met in person – faltering as I introduced myself and my research, and sensing that I was not engaging my audience. But after introducing some carefully chosen extracts from a moving novel about friendship, cancer and grief, I found myself listening to the group discussing in detail, without reservation, their wishes for their funerals and burials. Not only were fictional stories giving me a way of raising specific subjects and questions, but they were also helping me to encourage intimacy and establish trust within the virtual spaces. The environment of the online meetings could be changed by bringing stories into it. I could lead the participants towards laughter, tears, anger, confessions. Once again, the power of stories and the value of borrowed stories came to light.

During this period of intense research, in which I was usually working collaboratively with other people, I did not often have time to step back and reflect on what I was gaining from these experiences. I knew that I was privileged to witness other cancer patients telling their stories and responding to my ideas, but I did not spend time considering how this privilege might be shaping my own story. As I no longer had to contend with treatment and felt healthy and energetic, I was able to pursue my research goals with a focus and intensity that did not leave space for quiet, private thought. The world of academia seems to draw people into single-minded, obsessional patterns of life and thought, and this is what happened to me.

However, once I had made it through the pandemic, two things arrived in my life that forced me to step back and look again at my own story. The first of these major, life-changing developments was the return of romance to my story: the thrilling, joyful arrival of love in my life. During the lockdowns, the virtual meetings of an artistic group that I was part of had given me the chance to meet an enchanting, fascinating woman. Her capacity for creating beauty, and her love of nineteenth-century literature, when allied to an elegant, ethereal beauty, were irresistible. This wonderful woman, Karlee, turned out to be just as delightful in person as her virtual presence suggested she would be. And as soon as we met, I was lost – hopelessly, irretrievably in love. The suddenness and strength with which these feelings took hold of me was surprising. At this point, it was six years since I was first diagnosed with cancer and told that I had a fifty percent chance of living for more than five years. But I had not spent time considering passing this milestone and still saw romance as something that I was somehow distanced from because of my illness. This sense of uncertainty and caution was not enough to diminish my desire to spend time with Karlee, however, and we quickly became close. As our bond strengthened and an exciting intimacy developed, I began to realise that I was ready to brave the world of love and relationships again. The thinking and talking that I had devoted several years to, had been preparing me for this rediscovery of romance.

When the right moment came, I felt able to bare my soul and speak candidly about my physical, mental and emotional vulnerabilities. And Karlee reciprocated, telling me her own story of loss. I saw how exchanging stories can become the foundation of a strong, loving and honest romantic relationship. I learned more about the power of storytelling to create connection at the deepest levels. This meant that when Karlee and I eventually became a couple we both entered into the relationship in full awareness of the stories that we were becoming part of. She understood that she was likely to be a character who featured in the final chapters of my life, and I knew that I was joining Karlee in a season of grieving, recovering and rebuilding. I already knew, thanks to my family, the joy of entrusting my story to another person and knowing it was heard and respected. But in Karlee I had found a new person to place this trust in. Encouraged by her talent, intelligence and beauty, this surging joy quickly took the form of love. I could start to see everything that I had experienced before as a prelude: the precursor to a new chapter that was breath-taking in its unexpected delights.

A summer of picnics, idling and companionship followed as Karlee and I took advantage of the easing of COVID restrictions. Karlee's company was so distracting and comforting that, unwittingly, I started to slip back into a state of naive complacency as the future began to glow with promise. We talked often about the possibility of my cancer returning in lethal form, but this threat started to seem increasingly abstracted from the love and happiness at the heart of my story.

In this state of rosy joyfulness, it felt natural to both of us to intertwine our stories further. After careful thought, and consultation with loved ones, I proposed during a holiday on the Isle of Skye. Because I had been able to tell Karlee my story, I knew that – when she agreed to marry me – she understood what she was entering. Through exchanging stories, we had formed a bond strong enough to be tested in wholehearted commitment.

What I did not know was that a terrifying, heartbreaking challenge – the second life-changing development that would make me look again at my story – was about to arrive. Karlee had to endure the experience of promising to spend her life with me only to learn a few months later that she would soon have to watch me die. To indulge in melodrama while writing about this would not do justice to the calm courage with which she faced this shocking news. Many memories from the last year are raw and painful, but I will resist the temptation to wallow in sadness. We were engaged in September and in December I had an MRI scan: a routine six-month check-up. Because of complexities caused by COVID, I had arranged to hear the results of the scan via a phone call with my oncologist, expecting an easy conversation. But as soon as I heard my oncologist's voice, I could tell that our discussion would not be straightforward. She explained that the scans showed my tumour was growing again, expanding into new areas of my brain. The situation was dangerous and demanded urgent action. And, as my oncologist went on to tell me, I would have to return to treatment. Surgery would certainly be required, and this was likely to be followed by further treatment such as chemotherapy. I found my story changing once again; having been surprised by love and joy, I was now ambushed by tragedy.

This news was not only distressing because it announced disruption and suffering, but also because it undermined an illusion of safety and stability. This illusion had developed and strengthened over five years of clear scans, so it was well embedded. I am sure that I had inadvertently passed on some of the confidence and complacency it engendered in me to Karlee. So, both of us were shaken by the unexpected return of cancer and chaos. We were suddenly beset by practical problems: we would have to relocate at short notice and rearrange our lives around my illness and treatment. When writing about the impact of diagnosis on cancer patients, it might seem trivialising to focus on logistical issues. But, in my experience, it can be these smaller disturbances that prove most demoralising. To have to pack up our lives, having just arrived back at our home, while processing the news from my scans was almost too much to bear. To feel bereft of the time and peace to talk through the shock and sadness we felt was deeply dispiriting. All I wanted to do was to sit with Karlee and talk, weep, embrace. But I found myself cramming clothes into suitcases. As I cleared out the fridge, I reflected on our wedding plans, trying to work out if it was possible to organise a wedding while contending with cancer treatment. Loading files into boxes, I wondered about how many months I had left.

This question of 'how long' had become unavoidable since we learned of my cancer's return. We both knew that when a cancerous brain tumour reappears it is more likely to be aggressive and life threatening. The statistics suggested that death was now waiting in the next chapter of my life. But beginning a conversation about this, especially with those you love, is hard. There is never a good moment to start talking about death amid the rhythms of daily life. Space and tranquillity are vital starting points for painful discussions. We had to snatch brief, unsatisfactory pauses in the fraught packing process to start to talk through the implications of this plot twist. Dragging the focus of our attention away from marriage and romance, we began to pick through the debris of crushed dreams.

Yet this was when I began to borrow from Karlee's story, finding hope and resilience in her. This is not the place to tell her story, but I hope it is enough for me to say it is a tale of courage, dignity and principle shown in response to betrayal and cruelty. She is someone who never stops believing in, and fighting for, light, life and beauty. Her poise and bravery during times of turmoil tell a story of a remarkable 'inner baby': a soul shaped by an unquenchable commitment to goodness. This gave me a model to follow as I tried to re-imagine my own story once more. Like my family, Karlee made it easier to find fleeting moments of light in the swirling darkness, as well as helping me to hold fast to fortitude and faith. Her story contained a vision of emotional healing and recovery that resisted despair.

As we entered a phase of our lives that was – at times – almost comically strange and difficult, this vision guided and sustained me. After several meetings with oncologists and surgeons, it was decided that I should undergo brain surgery for a fourth time. The aim was to remove the tumour that was trespassing into new areas in my brain. Thankfully, new technology meant this could be done safely without me being kept awake during the procedure. But there was an added layer of complications caused by the COVID pandemic. Little details were different: masks, forms, hand sanitiser, distancing. But there was one particular difference that was especially difficult for me and my loved ones: I could have no visitors after the surgery. The idea of my recovery being a solitary time was distressing to me as well as to Karlee and my family. Being kept apart at a time when the comfort of closeness is so important was a frightening prospect. The surgeon did a superb job, removing all the tumour threatening my brain. But the recovery in hospital was a traumatic experience. I had been warned before the surgery that I was likely to find my speech function affected, as the procedure would cause swelling in my brain around the areas controlling speech. However, I had not anticipated how problematic this would be. I have always suffered from severe nausea after general anaesthetic, and this surgery was no exception. When I woke up, I felt extremely unwell: nauseous, weak and disorientated. As I slowly regained consciousness and began to understand my surroundings, I realised that I was in a busy, understaffed hospital ward. In this frenetic environment, patients were constantly arriving having just undergone surgery. The nursing staff, depleted due to COVID cases, were struggling to keep up with the stream of new arrivals and had little time to care for those already in the ward. Overcome with nausea, I was desperate for help. But due to my speech problems I struggled to make myself heard or understood as overworked nurses rushed past my bed.

I have never felt more keenly aware of my dependence and vulnerability as a patient. Nauseous, incoherent and afraid, I needed the kind of focused, attentive care that the nurses – through no fault of their own – could not give. In the past, this is where kind friends and family have intervened. As visitors on the ward, they had given me the personal care that I needed as I recovered from surgery. But the bizarre, unprecedented context of COVID had robbed me of this. Like so many other elderly, infirm or disabled people during the pandemic, I was lost in a care system that seemed to have no time for me. In the strange, stifling environment at the ward, I became increasingly confused. My attempts to ask for a sick bucket went unnoticed. I lost track of time, so that Karlee had to tell me via text message what day it was.

Looking back, I feel a tentative, strange gratitude for this harrowing experience. In part, because it made the joy of returning to home and family so much more intense. Yet also because my lonely recovery helped me to see how lost and rootless I would be without those people who have been alongside me during life with cancer. From their selves and stories, I have borrowed perseverance, resilience and hope. Whatever courage and determination have grounded me came from them. In hospital, distanced from Karlee and family, I was a solitary soul stripped of the support that I have always relied on.

Ewan was unable to complete his memoir before his death in December 2022. When he realised he was running out of time, he wrote the following conclusion reflecting on how he imagined hopeful futures for those he was leaving behind. These words have been transcribed from his notebook here.

Since then, I have needed that support more than ever. While the surgery was successful, it revealed that my cancer had become more aggressive. The prognosis for a patient in this position is very poor, so I know that I am probably living my final few months of life. That these months have included a punishing course of chemotherapy, more radiotherapy and several seizures has not made my transition to a terminal cancer patient easier. Feelings of grief and despair have been accompanied by nausea, pain and exhaustion. I have found myself reflecting on the things that I will leave behind when I die: people, ideas, writing, memories. The stinging sadness of death is tempered by these thoughts of a legacy – the sense that my death could be a form of beginnings, even a creative foundation.

I know that my spirit[16] in the world will be protected by those who have been part of my story. I have confidence in their ability to find joy and possibility in my death. I can sense that my research, reflection and time spent with other patients have all enabled me to approach death with peace. Through listening to other stories, I have learned to treat this final chapter as one that can contain beginnings, novelty and promise. I imagine rich, fulfilling futures flowing out of my ending.

One person in particular has helped me reach this point of peace. Just as I began to try to reconcile myself to death, my sister Laura was emerging from a time of loss and chaos. But she was not simply a survivor of tragedy. She had, throughout the turmoil, retained a clear sense of her right to justice and happiness. As a result she had found, during COVID, a difficult divorce and postnatal depression, a new life. Somehow she had endured and, ultimately, flourished.

A caring, steadfast husband, two charming children and a highly successful career were the fruit of her endurance and determination. By refusing to allow despair or self-pity to take hold, she made a time in which she witnessed the death of plans and aspirations into the beginning of a new chapter. The passion and commitment with which Laura confronts life, as well as her many gifts, have always inspired me. In this instance, she helped me to see that light and life can always be wrestled out of the grip of darkness. Through her example I saw clearly that setbacks and losses can always be reframed and transformed.

Laura's story may be the final one that I borrow from. It feels fitting that the end of my story should be shaped by a defiant, imaginative perspective borrowed from another person. As I think about death, legacy and those I leave behind, I understand that I am a composite: a synthesis of influences and stories. My sense of dependence and love for those I leave behind grows every day. With these reflections to comfort me, I am ready for my story to draw to a close.

PART II

Chapter 1
RETHINKING SPIRITUAL CARE

Ewan's overall introduction to his work 'From Beaune to *Breaking Bad*: Using the Arts to Meet Cancer Patients' Need and Desire for Spiritual Care'

Delivering spiritual care used to be more straightforward. In pre-Enlightenment Europe, spirituality was a relatively fixed concept, and linked to a predominantly Christian worldview. Healthcare institutions were familiar with this shared spirituality and knew how to cater for it, so those fortunate enough to receive care typically found that their spiritual needs were addressed, as well as their physical symptoms. In the famous *Hospices de Beaune*, founded in 1443, spirituality was integral to the care offered to the sick and dying. Staffed by a religious order, the hospice was intended to meet the medical and spiritual needs of patients, giving us a powerful example of the 'spiritual heritage' of nursing.[17] This dedication to the preservation and elevation of souls was symbolised in vibrant visual imagery by the Beaune Altarpiece. An ornate polyptych created by Rogier van der Weyden, the altarpiece consisted of a series of panels showing scenes from Christian hagiography. Saint

Sebastian and Saint Anthony, both associated with healing, were included in a range of images intended to reassure patients and direct their hearts and minds away from failing bodies towards higher things.[18]

By contrast, in modern, secular healthcare institutions like the NHS, such an approach to spiritual care is no longer viable. In part, this is because the vocabulary and practices of contemporary Western medicine are not well suited to dealing with spiritual concerns. The scientific revolution which began in the nineteenth century led medicine towards a 'new, unequivocal language of science' which 'spoke uniformly with neither time nor patience for narrative, poetry or paradox'.[19] What has become apparent, however, is that a language stripped of these qualities can describe a disease but cannot address a person. Carers have begun to realise that experiences and feelings related to spirituality, such as despair or hope, are not easy to engage with in the 'language of science'.[20] In an increasingly diverse and secular patient body, however, scenes of Christian salvation have simply lost their relevance and power: 'spirituality' is now a complex, contested idea that means different things to different people. Before we can even begin trying to 'do' spiritual care today, therefore, we must work out what spirituality might mean within this contemporary context. But is it even possible to establish a fixed definition of spirituality that accommodates atheists, agnostics, a plurality of religious traditions, and all the personal spiritualities that fall between these categories?

Considering this, it might be tempting to abandon the enterprise of spiritual care altogether. This is not, however, a reasonable option. A growing body of evidence informs us that patients both want and need spiritual care.[21] Patients still feel that spiritual issues are relevant to them, even if one person's idea of what these issues are may differ from another's. Although attempts have been made to design ways of addressing spiritual needs and delivering spiritual care, these have been hampered by uncertainty caused by the vagueness and subjectivity of spirituality today. As a result, spiritual care tends to be limited to a single question on a hospital admission form.[22] Important questions remain unanswered. What should spiritual care look like in the context of contemporary Western healthcare? How should it be delivered? And can the arts continue to play a role in the provision of spiritual care?

I want to show how accessible, popular artforms can play a vital role in this kind of care, filling the space left by the widespread move away from religious beliefs and practices in contemporary western society. Where once the intricate panels of the Beaune Altarpiece helped suffering souls to find consolation, I believe modern, mass-media artforms can enrich a cancer patient's search for meaning. Accessible fictional narratives found in novels, films, or television series often deal directly with the 'Big Questions' cancer raises, addressing themes like mortality, hope, and despair. These cultural products also tend to engage with the diverse, democratised form of spirituality prevalent in the arts today – the collective search for meaning amidst the chaos of life, sickness, and death.[23]

As such, these artforms can fulfil a role like religious symbolism and mythology, providing inspiration, stories, and imagery that can be integrated into care. The right novel, film or television series can be used to start the empathetic and imaginative conversations which should form the foundations of good spiritual care.[24] Art therapy techniques involving patients creating visual art – such as paintings or sketches – to express their spiritual concerns are already a tried and tested form of holistic care, but these alone are not enough.[25] Discussion of art and spiritual care needs to be expanded to include the forms of art people most frequently choose to engage with. For patients who are too ill, weary, or uncertain to create a piece of art capturing their thoughts and feelings, an accessible, engaging popular artwork can do this work for them: offering something to support spiritual exploration and reorientation.

I want my work to form a proposal, with supporting evidence, for a new way of understanding and doing spiritual care. As well as discussing why we need this, and how to understand the need, I'm going to use case studies to show what I mean.

In these case studies, I use one or two popular novels, films or television series as illustrative examples of artworks that address cancer patients' experiences. Each case study is focused on one of the four key areas of experience: time, mortality, humour, and sentimentality. These studies show how a range of different genres and media, such as 'tearjerker' novels, comedy films, and television dramas can present affirming, revealing portrayals of life with cancer. Moreover, the case studies describe in detail how the unique qualities of these different media afford specific things to cancer patients. It is not only that the narratives and characters may reflect a real patient's experiences in illuminating ways. The scope of a longform television drama, the language in a novel, or the audio-visual imagery in a film, for instance, can each invite a beholder to inhabit new perspectives on cancer, testing out alternative ways of understanding the disease and its impact. This can be thought-provoking, inspiring and liberating for patients searching for meaning. The artworks chosen for these case studies are representative of the depth of imaginative resources available 'out there'. In each case study, I refer to several other accessible, engaging artworks that address the theme in question, offering examples of what these might afford to someone affected by cancer. These examples are indicative of wider possibilities, showing how a single artwork might draw someone into a search for meaning supported and enriched by an array of creative, fictional responses to cancer in contemporary culture.

Responding to novels, films and television series in light of their personal experiences of cancer, people I worked with in discussion and focus groups were moved to re-evaluate their own life with cancer by an artwork, revealing the profoundly positive results this form of spiritual care can have. Participants also found affirmation in stories and imagery that captured their thoughts and feelings, discovering the 'language' for conveying their spiritual state that contemporary healthcare does not provide. Their voices show the tangible impact that arts-based spiritual care can have on patients' lives.

Here's how my argument runs in the rest of this book. In chapter two, I describe the problems in contemporary healthcare that have created a need for new forms of spiritual care. The emphases within modern medicine on objectivity, clinical science and empirical data have left little room for patients' personal, subjective spiritual concerns to be addressed. I also explain how the difficulties in defining spirituality hamper the provision of spiritual care, which is intended to address neglected areas of patients' experiences. However, I argue that a pragmatic understanding of spiritual care, intended to accommodate each patient's unique perspective, offers a viable solution to these difficulties. Finally, I describe how popular, accessible artworks can be used to frame a specific area of experience for cancer patients, providing material for reflection and discussion, whilst offering language, imagery and ideas for patients to draw on.

Then I address the theme of time, and the capacity for fictional narratives to reflect and re-frame cancer patients' experiences of time. My third chapter draws out three specific aspects of patients' experiences of time: a sense of 'lost time'; the unfamiliar and restrictive routines of cancer treatment; and the feeling of being trapped in an interminable cycle of suffering that many patients describe. Whilst outlining these areas of experience from a patient's perspective, I also show how these specific experiences are reflected in two fictional accounts of life with cancer: John Green's *The Fault in Our Stars*, and Alexander Solzhenitsyn's *Cancer Ward*. These novels reveal how cancer can disrupt and transform a patient's relationship to time resonating with real patients' experiences of 'days of absolutely nothing', or delays that 'seemed like forever'.

In chapter four, I use the television series *Breaking Bad* to illustrate how longform television drama can support a cancer patient's search for meaning in suffering and death. *Breaking Bad* is one of the many influential, accessible modern artworks that address the unsettling presence of death within a society often unwilling to confront human transience. I want to show how the series captures and conveys the isolation, anxiety or frustration that many cancer patients feel when suddenly made aware of their transience. I believe the series can also be used to invite patients to explore and discuss crucial, neglected issues, such as the balance between quality and quantity of life.

Chapter five is about something that might surprise people thinking about dealing with cancer: humour. It highlights the potential value of amusing, entertaining films about cancer for spiritual care. I explain how popular, accessible comedy films can be used to introduce cancer patients to the therapeutic or transformative impact of levity and laughter. I focus on a popular comedy film about cancer, *The Bucket List*, to reveal how accessible comic artworks can reframe cancer patients' experiences. *The Bucket List* features fictional illustrations of the capacity for humour to afford relief, hope, and truth for those affected by cancer. My research showed me how cancer patients' perspectives on cancer and humour were changed through watching and discussing these comedy films. There are risks but I argue that there is a way of integrating comedy films into 'humorous interventions' for cancer patients.

In chapter six, I present a new approach to the 'problem of sentimentality' in cancer care and contemporary culture. I want to show people shouldn't be too hostile towards what they see as 'sentimentality'. Cancer patients' testimonies and my own experience reveal that there are circumstances in which emotional experiences that might be deemed 'sentimental' can be valuable for those in need of respite or release. I look at two popular artworks about cancer seen as 'sentimental' by critics: Elizabeth Berg's novel *Talk Before Sleep*, and series 8 of the long-running television dramedy *Cold Feet*. I believe responses I have seen towards them show that – in the right moment – an accessible, sentimental artwork can meet a cancer patient's deepest needs.

Chapter 2
SPIRITUAL CARE AND THE ARTS

Trying to care for the 'spiritual self' involves vague, elusive concepts like love and art, which will mean different things to different patients. Yet this is exactly why the arts are an appropriate resource for spiritual care.[26] For instance, it is possible to assert with some confidence that Fyodor Dostoevsky's novel *The Idiot* will prompt a reader to reflect on sickness, death, and existential tumult, rather than hamsters or popcorn, yet this aspect is balanced by the fact that each person is free to respond to the presentation of these themes in their own way.[27]

As well as benefiting patients, using the arts to map out central themes in the experience of cancer can help carers with the problem of how best to 'initiate clear, meaning-centred conversations around the impact of diagnosis'.[28] Without training, support, or additional resources, it can be very difficult to know how best to broach such emotionally charged, sensitive subjects. A work of fiction offers a place for conversations to start, giving impetus, inspiration, and a framework for the exploration of a specific theme. Carers also report that, when trying to deliver spiritual care, it is often the case that approaching the topic directly was not seen as helpful amongst patients,[29] and artworks afford a means of opening up an area of experience for discussion in a sensitive, indirect manner, leaving patients free to refer to their own condition if and when they choose.

There have already been some small-scale attempts to test the impact of using the arts in Oncology Care. For instance, a one-off event for breast cancer survivors combining exhibitions, classes and leaflets aimed to demonstrate how '[a]rt can capture the most intimate and personal aspects of the cancer experience', and 'elicit significant emotional responses'.[30] A few of those writing about spiritual care mention anecdotal evidence indicating that using poetry or music to initiate discussion of spiritual concerns can have 'exceptionally positive' results, although they also acknowledge a lack of detailed research in this area.[31] Others point to progress made in art therapy techniques, suggesting this can 'enliven conversation', or 'bring illustrative examples' into play.[32] There is some evidence indicating that art therapy can be a useful tool for 'allowing cancer patients to express hidden emotions'.[33] However, this places significant demands on both carer and patient, requiring the therapist to provide materials and guidance, whilst also asking the patient to find ways of producing artworks which capture their innermost feelings, despite whatever mental or physical suffering they might be enduring.[34] There is still much debate concerning forms of art therapy involving the patient in 'visual art-making'.[35] Therapy in which carers must be instructed to 'remind the patients to enjoy the process',[36] and which relies upon the creation of profound, expressive artworks by severely ill patients, can cause anxiety,[37] and will have a limited application despite its clear value in some instances. Using existing, popular artworks to raise specific themes, opening a relevant area of experience for conversation, can provide an alternative option which avoids these problems.

Clinicians treating an illness do not simply declare that 'medicine could help'; they prescribe an appropriate remedy to be administered in a precise way, mindful of the context of the patient and their condition. If artworks are to be used in a targeted way to open up spiritual areas of experience, encourage conversation, and introduce illustrative examples, this must be done in a careful, considered manner. Rather than treating the arts as equivalent to a prescribed clinical treatment, a methodology that recognises the depth and complexity of an artwork must be followed. Matters of personal taste, cultural preference and interpretation will also need to be considered.

And when it comes to what I'm calling 'the arts' or 'culture', I mean that in its widest sense, embracing everything that patients might come across. Since the turn of the century, millions of people have read John Green's novel *The Fault in Our Stars* (2012), about love, cancer, art, and spirituality. Tens of millions have watched several series of *Breaking Bad* on Netflix (2008-2013), a direct, uncompromising exploration of the existential turmoil cancer can cause. Many more of the most successful films, television series and novels of recent times, such as *Fargo* (2014-), *Cold Feet* (2016-), *A Monster Calls* (2011), *The Bucket List* (2008), *Catastrophe* (2015-2019), *Orange is the New Black* (2013-2019), *Mad Men* (2007-2015), *After Life* (2019-), *Talk Before Sleep* (1994), *The Fault in Our Stars* (2012), *The Kominsky Method* (2018-), and *Deadpool* (2016) have dealt in detail with the impact of cancer upon peoples' lives.[38] These artworks are bringing the 'big questions' cancer raises to the foreground, so studying how they achieve this, and how people respond, will give vital information about the interrelation of cancer, art and spirituality.

And in what follows I'm using not only my own experience as a cancer patient but also what I learned from others in two particular research projects where I tested some of my ideas and listened to what other patients made of them. I used two qualitative research projects to test out my arts-based approach to spiritual care in practice. The intention was to show how the approach outlined in this chapter can inform the design of effective, practical spiritual care resources for cancer patients. I trialled two new care resources: a 'Fiction Library' resource and a series of guided group discussions. These trials formed part of research collaborations with Maggie's Cancer Care Centres and the Northumberland Cancer Support Group (NCSG).[39] My work with the patients, friends and family, staff, psychologists, and cancer support specialists involved with these charities shaped the development of my research project.

One source of the empirical evidence presented in this thesis was a series of focus groups, facilitated by Maggie's and NCSG. These were designed to examine whether popular novels, films, and television series could facilitate and enhance a dynamic, communal exploration of salient spiritual themes. Results suggested this can be an effective way of generating empathetic communication, giving people a valuable opportunity to disclose their cancer story. In the groups, extracts from a novel, film, or television series were used to initiate reflection and conversation, addressing a specific area of experience. This provided a 'way into' subjects that might otherwise be too sensitive or distressing to address, offering participants a means of speaking indirectly about personal experiences, whilst hearing others' perspectives. Evidence from the groups demonstrated that this can be a revealing and uplifting process for patients, affording affirmation and insight to those involved. Moreover, holding several virtual focus groups provided evidence of the capacity for popular artworks to facilitate discussion, foster community and enhance mutual understanding amongst members of support groups when meeting in-person is impossible.

The results of these qualitative research projects should not of course be considered a representative study. However, 30 participants recruited through two separate cancer support charities, and from several different locations across the United Kingdom, were enough to produce responses informed by a wide range of experiences and perspectives. As the evidence presented in later chapters will show, the ways in which participants were affected by the artworks investigated in this project were personal, and often contrasting, due to the unique circumstances of the individuals involved. Although the nature of the research meant that I needed to keep patients' views anonymous, I've woven their thoughts and opinions into what I'm now going to explore.

Chapter 3
CANCER, TIME AND FICTION

John Green's bestselling novel *The Fault in Our Stars* is an excellent example of what popular, mass-media artworks can offer a cancer patient in need of spiritual care. One of the most widely read explorations of the problem of suffering ever written, Green's young adult novel has become arguably the most famous fictional exploration of living with cancer.[40] *The Fault in Our Stars* is a search for spiritual nourishment amidst stretches of time disrupted or truncated by cancer. Green spent ten years working on the novel after leaving his position as chaplain at a children's hospital ministering to young patients and their families. Overwhelmed by what he encountered in the hospital, Green says he 'found the experience almost too sad to bear'.[41] Before taking up the post, Green had studied religion and literature, but he explains that the 'fancy theological ideas from reading lots of theological books didn't really matter much when it came to being with kids who were dying'.[42] Yet rather than abandoning the subject, Green says he left the hospital wanting to 'write a novel about sick kids',[43] conceiving *The Fault in Our Stars* as a means of 'trying to understand some of the ways through that [experience]'.[44]

In turning to popular fiction to find meaning in his traumatic tenure as a hospital chaplain, Green set himself apart from many influential theological responses to cancer.[45] Green sought out a wider audience and a new medium. Consequently, *The Fault in Our Stars* is a fictional narrative that can afford affirmation and inspiration to cancer patients with diverse spiritual perspectives, as they contend with the power of cancer to dictate and damage lives. Both cancer patients and caregivers have specifically identified *The Fault in Our Stars* as a novel that can accurately reflect real experiences of cancer.[46]

In this chapter I want to show how two fictional narratives – John Green's *The Fault in Our Stars* and Alexander Solzhenitsyn's *Cancer Ward* – can provide spiritual resources to cancer patients whose sense of time has been changed by what they are going through. Both novels deal directly, and in detail, with human experiences of life with cancer. Each offers a range of interesting perspectives on the significance of time within these experiences, and on the role that reading fiction can play in transforming patients' sense of time. Alongside his difficult, brief ministry as a hospital chaplain, a major influence on the development of *The Fault in Our Stars* was Green's friendship with Esther Earl, a young woman who died of cancer aged sixteen.[47] Green credited Earl with teaching him that 'a short life can be a good life, a full life', implying that this relationship influenced his conception of time as he worked on *The Fault in Our Stars*.[48] Meanwhile, Solzhenitsyn wrote *Cancer Ward* having experienced a tortuous wait for surgery on a tumour whilst in prison camp.[49] The experience of enduring delays, even as he felt a cancerous tumour growing within him, evidently provided impetus when it came to creating a fictional examination of the impact of cancer upon a patient's sense of time. *The Fault in Our Stars* and *Cancer*

Ward are therefore especially apposite works for supporting an argument in favour of using literary narratives to open up and explore the theme of time. An unlikely dialogue between the literature of Green and Solzhenitsyn provides fascinating examples of the ways in which fictional narratives can help cancer patients rediscover a more positive, personal and nourishing relationship with all things temporal.

I'll also explain how cancer patients may experience time, drawing out three issues which are repeatedly raised by those living with cancer: a sense of 'lost time' and disrupted plans; unfamiliar, unforgiving medical regimens; and a sense of being trapped in an interminable cycle of suffering. Then I'll explain how these fictional stories can also help patients to escape problematic thought patterns and to reshape their relationships to time, capturing their personal experiences in a manner that rigid, clinical 'clock time' cannot.

Alan Lewis, in his theological examination of time, cancer and existential tumult, argues that the long stretches of 'inertia' involved in cancer treatment force 'contemporary Westerners' to face their 'fear of time's expanses'. The contrast between the 'frantic pace' of modern life, and the 'stasis' which can characterise life with cancer, brings a new awareness of the 'power of time to tease us'.[50][51] For instance, describing what they believed that *The Fault in Our Stars* could afford a cancer patient struggling to process their experiences, one participant in my focus groups said: 'it's important when you're going through something like this, to know that you're not the only one'. They argued that reading Green's novel could provide this affirmation, adding: 'to read *The Fault in Our Stars* like this, I would think for anyone that's having trouble reconciling themselves with what they're going through this would be extremely helpful'.[52]

Green employs an informal, intimate first-person

narrative voice that encourages readers to identify and sympathise with the novel's main character.[53] Meanwhile, Solzhenitsyn's narrative grants the reader access to the interior monologues of several different residents of the cancer ward, offering a range of perspectives for readers to inhabit. So both novels invite a reader to relate to characters who are finding their sense of time reshaped by cancer, presenting voices that might capture aspects of real patients' experiences

Being diagnosed with cancer is invariably a shocking, unsettling experience, and patients often describe this in terms of a changing attitude towards time. Carers note that when a patient is told that cancer may cut short their life, 'time for him [or her] gains a completely different meaning'.[54] Therapists also observe that a disease which brings a heightened awareness of the 'imminence of death' will often 'affect profoundly a person's experience of time and space'.[55] Kübler-Ross provides the example of an interview with a patient who is determined to defy her prognosis in order to care for her two sons. The patient insists that 'we all have a time to go and it's not my time', as she is desperate to be 'saved just long enough to raise these boys'.[56] Time, and how much she had left, became a source of uncertainty and apprehension for this patient, and she is not an isolated case; a study of the impact of a breast cancer diagnosis on patients found that the discovery was perceived as causing 'a multitude of smaller deaths that relate to the hopes, dreams, expectations and possibilities' of those affected.[57]

Readers of Solzhenitsyn's *Cancer Ward* are left in no doubt as to this power of cancer to distort and disrupt a patient's sense of time. Solzhenitsyn's character, the student Vadim, helpfully exemplifies a certain way of approaching cancer and time.[58] Cancer has reshaped his attitude, causing him to feel disdain for 'anything which is not 'time usefully spent''. Solzhenitsyn invites the reader into Vadim's frantic thoughts, and his fury about 'unfinished work', 'interrupted interests' and 'unfulfilled opportunities' following his diagnosis. Vadim's desire to become a 'doctor of science' despite his 'death sentence' has left him gripped by 'a demonic, insatiable hunger for time'.[59] Just as Kübler-Ross's patient is desperate for 'just long enough' to raise her children, so Vadim's life becomes a restless race against the clock. For patient and fictional character alike, time is to be fought and resisted: an obstacle which causes only anger and apprehension.[60]

Gus, Hazel's love interest in The Fault in Our Stars, clearly feels the 'hunger for time' which grips Solzhenitsyn's Vadim. He describes life with cancer as like 'Russian roulette' and vents his frustration over time-consuming treatments: 'I was going through hell for six months ... then at the end, it still might not work'.[61] Like Vadim, Gus's character provides insight into the perception of 'time being lost' which medical literature connects to cancer, illustrating the overwhelming patterns of thought this can set in motion. Meanwhile, Hazel's experiences of waiting in hospital, enduring 'undays of staring at acoustic ceiling tile and watching television and sleeping and pain and wishing for time to pass',[62] resonated with several participants in the focus groups. One participant recognised the 'days of absolutely nothing' that feel like 'a complete waste' that Green describes whilst another said that the passage reminded them of the 'time between having my second and third chemotherapy, that seemed like forever'.

Frustration at lost time can be exacerbated by hospital treatments. When the symptoms of disease, and side-effects of treatments and medications, are combined with the hospital environment, Lewis describes the result as a 'heart-breaking routine of monotonous misery'.[63] For instance, the schedule for radiotherapy usually begins with 'an anxious delay for patients before treatment', followed by a 'daily wait for several days or weeks' once radiation begins.[64] All of this also takes place in surroundings which are not well equipped for returning a patient to a more positive, secure relationship to time. A cancer ward is an 'alien' world for patients: an environment that can 'turn night into day' and 'clash with regular life'.[65] For someone recuperating after surgery, radiotherapy or chemotherapy, the healing familiarity of natural circadian rhythms is overridden by frequent injections, doses and check-ups which draw attention to the 'cruel rhythms of bodily dysfunction'.[66][67]

In *Cancer Ward*, Solzhenitsyn captures the unease and trepidation these 'cruel rhythms' cause in the ward, by structuring whole chapters around the consultants' rounds. As they travel between the beds, the clinicians bring a 'wave of attention, fear and hope' wherever they go, whilst they discuss 'sessions' for treatment schedules. In the chapter entitled 'The patients' worries', the narrative focus switches between the residents of the ward while they wait to be assessed, following the clinical team around. One patient sits with a 'tense expression', watching for the team's arrival, and another 'kept a sharp look out' for the doctors, and 'had been getting himself ready for some time' when they finally reached him.[68] The nervous energy which pervades the chapter reflects the tension and apprehension felt by real patients, whose lives are shaped by these anxiety-inducing routines.

Similarly, in *The Fault in Our Stars*, the narrative becomes a means of illuminating the disruptive influence of these routines. Green uses the striking image of a small oxygen tank, which Hazel must always drag behind her, to illustrate the way the demands of treatment can restrict patients' lives. The tank needs refilling regularly, and this imposes a controlling schedule onto all Hazel does, becoming one of her character's distinctive features.[69] The process of setting up the tank and its timings is woven into the narrative alongside dialogue and plot developments, influencing each of these. When a poignant, emotional exchange between Hazel and her mother is interrupted by this process – 'she set it for 2.5 litres a minute – six hours before I'd need a change'[70] – it is redolent of the 'heart-breaking routines of monotonous misery', and 'wearing in-out timetables' referred to in patient testimonies.[71]

The overall effect of these negative experiences – feelings of lost time, disrupted plans and life-limiting regimes – can be an impression of endless suffering. Patients can reach a point at which 'languor settles in', when time starts to feel 'static' and 'flattens out into a perpetual present'.[72] Trying to express this bleak prospect, a cancer patient in art therapy drew a series of circles, containing the words 'circles, circles, going round in circles... Is there any way out of this maze?'. The result was a 'powerful image of frustration at the repetitive, unending nature' of treatment.[73] As Lewis observes, this cry for a 'way out' reveals how the experience of cancer can appear to promise only 'seeming aeons of nausea and wretchedness', to be tolerated 'without any guarantee of a future to hang on for'.[74]

All this shows patients urgently searching for ways of doing justice to troubling experiences, and it is these imaginative tools which literary art can supply. The sense of an interminable struggle with cancer is mirrored in the two novels in question. Solzhenitsyn develops Vadim's character to reflect this, allowing his 'tightly strung capacity for work', and belief there were 'not enough hours in the day' to be gradually worn down by the numbing ordeal of treatment. Eventually, the frenetic, ambitious doctoral researcher is left thinking that the hours were 'too long', because 'there was not enough life' to fill them.[75] This shift towards abject despair, embodied in the narrative's progression, captures the drastic perspective patients can ultimately reach.[76]

This portrayal of time spent in a cancer ward in terms of life-sapping perpetuity is very similar to Hazel's narration of her own stays in hospital in *The Fault in Our Stars*. Given direct access to her thoughts during these periods, the reader discovers that she began to feel like 'the subject of some existentialist experiment in delayed gratification'.[77] In a conversation with her oncologist, Hazel is told that her doctors have 'seen people live with your level of tumour penetration for a long time'. Yet this vague, jargonistic assessment causes only apprehension, surfacing unpleasant memories for Hazel: 'I did not ask what constituted a long time. I'd made that mistake before'.[78] This was also a passage that resonated with several participants in the focus groups. Identifying with Hazel, one participant described the passage as exposing 'the obvious difference between the professional view and their language, and what it's like to be a patient'. Observing that 'the fact that Hazel doesn't want to ask what constitutes a long time' reflects how such a discussion with an oncologist can be 'a very emotional experience for the patient', the participant contrasted Hazel's description of the meeting with the 'professional, medical language' used by physicians: 'it's almost as if they are talking about the same thing, but from two completely different perspectives'.

Another participant suggested that Hazel's lack of agency in the meeting reflected their own encounters with oncologists, saying: 'sometimes people [physicians] can just talk over you and then the meeting is finished'. Clearly, Hazel's position as a passive patient, receiving pronouncements on her remaining time delivered in opaque medical jargon, felt relatable to participants in the focus groups with direct experience of such meetings. Hazel's interior monologue, like Vadim's changing attitude towards the hours in a day, forms part of a detailed, thoughtful probing of how cancer could reshape a patient's attitude towards time. And for those confronted with this reality, discovering echoes of their experiences outside of private, undisclosed thoughts can help them to move towards acknowledging, understanding and expressing their changing relationship to time.[79]

However, this is not all that artworks can afford. Having introduced cancer patients to a world in which their experiences of time were affirmed and reflected in accessible, relatable characters and stories, fictional narratives can also offer new ways of perceiving these experiences. When a patient has become caught up in an angry, embittered struggle against the passage of time, those offering spiritual care will need to promote a 'different understanding of time'.[80] As palliative care consultant Dr Mark Taubert suggests, carers must try to give patients alternatives which enable them to step off the 'treadmill' of closed, calculated time. He argues that turning the 'kaleidoscope' through which time is seen can shift a patient's focus 'away from the numbers' and 'the change in the scans', allowing them to see time in a new, 'beautiful' light.[81] And fictional narratives can help cancer patients to access this beauty from beyond the boundaries of clock time.

This is directly relevant to cancer patients who urgently need to discover new perspectives on time. In *The Fault in Our Stars*, Hazel – an avid reader – is especially taken by one particular novel, *An Imperial Affliction*, which she describes as 'the closest thing I had to a Bible'.[82] It tells the story of a young girl who contracts blood cancer, and Hazel finds that the author 'seemed to understand [her] in weird and impossible ways'.[83] Searching for meaning in her own experiences of cancer, Hazel discovers a fictional voice which speaks directly to her own sense of self, whilst also introducing her to 'weird and impossible' ways of understanding her life. This is not a form of escapism, simply providing a distraction, but a narrative which sets Hazel free, allowing her to understand personal experiences in a new way.[84] Green's novel uses Hazel's formative relationship with her favourite novel to point to the power of literary fiction to cast difficult situations in a 'weird' light, thus making it possible to 'turn the kaleidoscope' and find beauty amidst the waves of suffering. *Cancer Ward* and *The Fault in Our Stars* each contain ideas which can bring about this shift in understanding, allowing patients to see the passage of time in a new light.

The imagery which literary fiction creates can provide flexible, fluid concepts of time that are 'indispensable' in the search for a new language to describe time's structures.[85] When Oleg, the main protagonist in *Cancer Ward*, is given a break from treatment and allowed to leave the hospital, his response illustrates the extent to which the meaning of time can shift dramatically for a cancer patient. Yet rather than regarding this distortion as a problem to be solved, Oleg embraces the fact that, suddenly, 'everything was new and had to be understood afresh'. As he strolls outside, Oleg feels as if it were 'the first day of his new life', reflecting that 'years of his life could not compare with today'.[86] Up to this point, Solzhenitsyn has described in detail Oleg and his fellow patients' residency in the cancer ward, using characters like Vadim to acknowledge that these periods can be filled with a sense of 'unfulfilled opportunities', or dominated by an 'insatiable hunger for time'. But here, Oleg's internal monologue reframes the preceding narrative, casting it as merely the prelude to a glorious 'today' suffused with 'early-morning springtime joy'.[87]

A cancer patient reading this passage will not find the difficult reality of treatment and hospital stays ignored, but will be offered a different way of addressing themselves to these experiences, focused on the promise of a more joyful 'today' to come.

This reveals how cancer's capacity to uproot a patient's sense of time could be regarded as an invitation, as well as a challenge. And The Fault in Our Stars also illustrates how this might become an opportunity to entertain more expansive and malleable concepts of time. David Brown argues that art can help its audience to explore 'the more 'open' universe of which contemporary science now speaks',[88] investigating a world in which, as Einstein claimed, 'the separation between past, present and future has the value of mere illusion'.[89] Green's novel can afford a cancer patient access to this more complex sense of time, encouraging them to reach beyond more restrictive perspectives. Returning from a romantic holiday, which has been tainted with tragedy by his admission that he is dying of cancer, Gus starts talking to Hazel about temporality. He tells her that, as they are in a 'superfast airplane', 'right now time is passing slower for us than for people on the ground'. Even better, this means he will 'live longer' during their journey, 'because of relativity or whatever'.[90] Patient testimony details how an 'awareness of the imminence of death' can 'affect profoundly' a cancer patient's sense of time and space,[91] but Gus's vocalised mental meanderings suggest that this reconceptualising can yield constructive results. Green's fiction implies that a cancer patient might allow the destabilising of their sense of time to draw them into this open universe of modern science, granting them opportunities to 'live longer' by refusing to be confined within the illusion of time ticking away in a regulated, unchanging fashion.[92]

The sources describing patient experience showed how the overall impact of cancer upon an individual's sense of time can lead patients to feel they are trapped within 'repetitive, unending' cycles of illness, treatment and recovery. Yet, as the narrative of *Cancer Ward* develops, this sense of repetitious, boundless torment is challenged. In amongst Vadim's convoluted reflections on time is a reference to Epicurus's observation that 'a fool, if offered eternity, would not know what to do with it'. For Vadim, Epicurean philosophising about a 'fool with eternity in hand' constitutes justification for his decision to 'dismiss all day-dreams of recovery or life prolonged' and work continuously on his doctorate.[93] However – through Vadim's reflections – Solzhenitsyn has slipped into the reader's mind the possibility that a notional 'eternity' spent on a cancer ward is something the patient can take 'in hand' and treat as space full of potential. The irony of Vadim's obsessional, single-minded use of his time will only strengthen a patient's suspicion that there may be other ways of looking at their own time with cancer.

In another of his novels, *The Gulag Archipelago*, Solzhenitsyn tells the story of an astronomer who – when he was made a political prisoner – found that 'counting the passing minutes put him intimately in touch with the universe'. The prisoner 'saved himself only by thinking of the eternal... and what Time and the passing of Time really are'. Imprisoned, and left to think, the astronomer treated this as an opportunity to re-evaluate the nature of Time itself, and consequently 'began to discover a new field in physics'.[94] In *Cancer Ward*, these different ways of 'thinking of the eternal' are also hinted at, as the reader is invited to look on unbounded periods of stillness as an invitation to consider what they could do with their own 'eternity in hand'.

There are also intimations of the positive potential of timelessness in *The Fault in Our Stars*. The epigraph to the novel, taken from the fictitious work *An Imperial Affliction*, is a metaphor of time as the tidal movement of an ocean 'rising up and down, taking everything with it' – a fluid entity that surges in cyclical patterns, revealing, shaping and concealing as it moves.[95] The idea of perpetuity is framed as a shifting tidal rhythm, rather than an endless stretch of one-directional duration.[96] Spiritual carers are tasked with becoming 'champions of a different understanding of time',[97] and Green's use of narrative sequence and metaphor shows one way in which this can be achieved. When the reader comes to reflect on Hazel and Gus's encounters with dragging stretches of time, this imagery has placed them in the position of Solzhenitsyn's astronomer, who is thinking of time and the eternal in novel, imaginative ways. And for a cancer patient, this can also provide them with a lens through which to re-examine their own relationship to time and timelessness.

In *Cancer Ward*, Solzhenitsyn manipulates the pace of his narrative to create luxurious, saturated spaces in time, which cut through clock-governed hospital timescales. The most celebrated instance of this is found in a scene in which Oleg is taken into a treatment room for a blood test. As the procedure begins, the rate of plot development decelerates, as intricate details take up increasing quantities of discursive space. Looking around him, Oleg sees 'the bottles of brown blood, the shining bubbles, the tops of the sunlit windows, the reflections of the windows with their six panes in the frosted glass', and finally 'the whole expanse of ceiling with its shimmering patch of sunlight'.[98] The swelling significance of intricacies fills a single instance with detail, arresting time's progression and checking its momentum. Michael Acoutrier describes this scene as 'beautiful precisely for its interminability'. The narrative progression is 'microscopic', and the cadence of the scene is 'deliberately retarded to allow the hero to savour the moment of relaxation, of peace, of repose'.[99] Natalie Weaver argues that it is important for spiritual care to help patients find meaning through 'centredness in the present', generating new feelings of 'energy and interest'.[100] The focus and immediacy of Solzhenitsyn's intensified moments, I would suggest, fashions an imaginative space in which a patient could practise such centredness. The familiar scenario of waiting while blood is taken or injected becomes a vastness to be savoured.

Recalling the patient who, after hearing his cancer diagnosis, saw 'every moment' as a living 'hell', it is tempting to wonder whether Solzhenitsyn's novel could allow a patient in this position to grasp more rewarding moments, set apart from anxious anticipation. *Cancer Ward* contains scenes in which 'moments are no longer just the stages of a struggle' and have become 'the pulsations of a return to life' instead.[101] After his death, Kalanithi's wife wrote of the 'simple moments' she had shared with her husband: moments 'swelled with grace and beauty' that provided solace amid sickness and chemotherapy.[102] It is these nourishing, life-giving spaces that a fictional narrative like *Cancer Ward* can encourage a cancer patient to seek out within their own lives, and to cherish as islands of timeless peace.

In *The Fault in Our Stars*, the language of infinities plays a crucial role in the portrayal of the lives of two young cancer patients. However, it is not primarily used for describing endless cycles of illness and treatment, but as a metaphor for time spent within a loving human relationship. In an analogous approach to *Cancer Ward*, Green's novel also asks the reader to realise that protracted moments of 'grace and beauty' can still form part of a life troubled by cancer. An important scene in *The Fault in Our Stars* sees Hazel, accompanied by Gus, meet the author of the novel which had become so important to her, *An Imperial Affliction*. The author, Van Houten, turns out to be a crushingly disappointing person: an arrogant, aloof drunkard who refuses to answer Hazel's questions. He insists his novel is 'an obvious and unambiguous metaphorical representation of God' and will not indulge Hazel's desire to know about the fate of the human characters 'independent of their metaphorical meanings or whatever'. However, during his unhelpful drunken ramblings, Van Houten inadvertently introduces Hazel and Gus to Zeno's 'tortoise paradox' regarding a runner trying to catch a tortoise who has a head start, expressing the idea that 'some infinities are bigger than other infinities'.[103]

Van Houten's attempt to steer their attention away from his novel accidently provides the two teenage lovers with a concept that will eventually deepen their understanding of the precious time they spent together. Later in the story, Hazel, recalling a memory shared with Gus, describes it as a 'brief but still infinite forever'.[104] A key claim in the theologian Richard Bauckham's work is that whilst 'art cannot conquer transience', it can 'give eternity a temporarily enduring place in time'.[105] Hazel's interpretation of her past in terms of transient infinites illustrates how Bauckham's idea could translate directly into human experience. As Hazel provides the narrative voice, we can see the notion of a fleeting forever influencing her thoughts and allowing her to express more fully what time with Gus has meant to her.

The significance of this is best understood by looking back at Hazel's previous relationship to time. I have already noted that Green describes her feeling like the subject of an 'existentialist experiment in permanently delayed gratification' whilst in hospital. And, in a separate conversation with her oncologists, we are also told about the sense of unease Hazel felt when discussing lengthy spells of time: 'I did not ask what constituted a long time. I'd made that mistake before'.[106] Yet after having met Gus, and discovered the idea of a brief infinity suffused with love, her attitude towards time's expanses is characterised by loving nostalgia, rather than cancer-caused distortion and deferment.[107] This discovery of newfound agency and empowerment can be crucial in a spiritual care context. NHS chaplain Christopher Swift argues that 'attention to language in health care settings' is vital. He suggests that studying this can 'reveal some of the implicit workings of power within an organisation', specifically words which cast a patient as a 'passive recipient of medical instruction' who must 'wait for new measurements of progress'.[108] When the reader first comes across Hazel, they find her a hostage to the language of long waits, and measurements of her oxygen tank's capacity. Yet as the narrative progresses, we are shown the emphasis gradually moving towards meanings which she shapes to fit her experiences of love and loss.

This really resonated with some participants in my focus groups. For one, Hazel's developing relationship to time reflected their own experiences. The participant said that 'when you're faced with something like cancer, your perception of time changes altogether', relating how the discussion of *The Fault in Our Stars* in the focus group had resonated with their belief that cancer can bring a 'totally different perspective on what is important'. Responding to this, another participant raised the issue of the impact of drugs and cancer treatments, weighed against the value of life. They noted that healthcare institutions assume that if a treatment 'is going to cost ten-thousand pounds a month, and it's just going to give people a few more months of life... it makes perfect economic sense not to be administered'. However, Hazel's reclaiming of the language of time, along with the discussion in the focus group, gave this participant a means of expressing their resistance to this medical monetisation of time.

'Hazel was talking about "a long time", and her idea of a long time was completely different to the medical idea of a long time. And I think unless you've been through what everybody in this meeting [the focus group] has been through, you can appreciate that a few months can be something absolutely magnificent, and not anything to be dismissed as unimportant. So, this whole meeting today has really reinforced that for me'.

Clearly, decisions about withholding treatment and financing medicines are complex and contested, and never taken lightly. Yet what Hazel's narrative voice appeared to offer participants is a means of conveying, powerfully and persuasively, their particular perspectives on time, inspiring their rejection of the role of a 'passive recipient of medical instruction'. Within the NHS, debates around the monetary value of a life, and the cost of life-prolonging treatments, are becoming increasingly significant as ever more sophisticated, effective treatments are developed.[109] As such, a fictional narrative that helps patients take a more active role in these debates, conveying the true value of their time, can be extremely important.

Describing an eleventh-hour reconciliation between a father dying of prostate cancer and his son, hospice chaplain Richard F. Groves describes a 'transcendent quality to the experience', which showed that when 'extreme spiritual pain is finally relieved, death opens onto a fulcrum of eternity'.[110] Speaking at Gus's funeral, Hazel gives a fictional echo of this experience: 'Gus, my love, I cannot tell you how thankful I am for our little infinity ... You gave me a forever within the numbered days.'[111] The 'spiritual pain' which Hazel had once associated with mentions of 'a long time' has gradually been assuaged, as the language of forever now evokes memories of her 'little infinity' with Gus. Viewed through the prism of loving relationships, time and transience can open onto a 'fulcrum of eternity'. Hazel's narrative eventually becomes an invitation to explore this possibility and to look on life with cancer through this new lens.[112]

Responding to this invitation, one participant in the focus groups argued that Hazel's words captured how a health crisis can change our relationship to time in constructive ways. They suggested her speech is relevant to 'any crisis in life' because 'that's how you face situations and use time'. Indeed, they believed that Hazel's speech conveyed the manner in which a health crisis 'arrests you and makes you think'. Another participant explained that they felt Hazel's eulogy had applications beyond their experiences of cancer, saying 'if I hadn't known it was about cancer, it could be about our COVID situation: it's about making the most of family, making the most of time and appreciating things'. Furthermore, a participant in the Fiction Library trial, when asked if any of the artworks had raised issues relevant to their experiences of cancer, identified *The Fault in Our Stars* as a novel that expressed the swelling significance of 'small pleasures' during their life with cancer. Writing that Green's novel captured 'the dual and seemingly contradictory elements of knowing one has – or expects to have – a shortened lifespan', the participant observed that 'in *The Fault in Our Stars* and *The Time Traveller's Wife*[113] there are numerous examples of small, simple pleasures taking on special significance when time together is condensed, tomorrow uncertain and now is all they have'. Explaining the value of this, the participant added that 'the gift/curse issue that I experienced [whilst living with cancer]' was revealed through these novels, as they seemed consonant with the sense of a shared pleasure expanding to hold 'special significance'. [114]

An interesting feature of Hazel's transition towards this deeper understanding of time is the role played by Van Houten, the fictional author, within it. His book may have been able to reflect Hazel's experience of cancer, echoing her thoughts in 'weird and impossible ways', but this is because of her personal response, rather than Van Houten's authorial intent.[115] Fascinatingly, the value of treating a fictional novel about cancer as open to a reader's personal engagement with the text, rather than discrete and closed off to new meanings, was illustrated in the response of one participant in the focus groups. They described how *The Fault in Our Stars* 'meant such a lot' to them, before explaining that they had also looked for *An Imperial Affliction*, wanting to purchase the novel, because 'it meant such a lot to Gus and Hazel that I wanted to... find out what it was'. When they discovered *An Imperial Affliction* was fictitious, they chose to buy a blank copy of this imaginary work online: 'I still wanted to have it even though it was empty, because... I thought that one day, I might want to write something in it'. Evidently, the participant perceived Green's work to be open to their personal ideas and experiences, treating the blank canvas of *An Imperial Affliction* as an invitation to self-expression. The physical space of the blank pages, ready to receive their thoughts and feelings, provided a symbol for the participant's constructive engagement with the meanings contained within Green's novel.

Green uses his fiction to deal directly with these important issues surrounding authorship, interpretation, and subjectivity. Instead of shying away from the fact that he is producing a piece of fiction that will likely elicit strong, profoundly personal feelings, he shows an awareness of what his artform leaves open to the reader.[116] The irreconcilability of Hazel and Van Houten's interpretations warns writers, critics and scholars that becoming wedded to preconceived ideas of how a book ought to be understood can cut them off from the immediacy and intimacy of subjective responses.[117] In a telling exchange of views, Van Houten ridicules Hazel for saying that *An Imperial Affliction* meant a great deal to her: 'what do you mean by *meant*? Given the futility of our struggles, is the fleeting jolt of meaning that art gives us valuable?'.[118] Green appears to be making two points here: firstly, the jolt of meaning art can provide is indeed valuable, and his novel is motivated by faith in this; secondly, what an artwork 'means' is not exclusively controlled by the author, as meaning is generated in the 'constructive engagement' between a reader and the text.

Conclusion

Using literary fiction to address cancer patients' spiritual pain, and change their relationship to time, is not a straightforward process. It is impossible to predict exactly what these fictional narratives will afford an individual patient. A novel may include details which do not ring true for a patient, conflicting with their feelings about living with cancer, or their taste in literature. It will also be likely that at various stages in the process of treatment and recovery, certain ideas, descriptions or characters will strike a patient in different ways, and their resonance and relatability will vary accordingly. However, these considerations also underline why fiction can be a valuable resource for cancer patients disturbed or frustrated by time. *Cancer Ward* and *The Fault in Our Stars* illustrate how a single narrative can hold together several voices or perspectives in creative tension. Solzhenitsyn's ward is crammed with human life in all its diversity. Several worldviews are conveyed and explored, and through this, many ways of relating to time. In *The Fault in Our Stars*, as the two protagonists navigate the challenges life with cancer presents, the reader is given privileged access to their evolving thought processes and shifting attitudes towards time. Because of this, both novels open a space which could accommodate a wide spectrum of views on cancer and time, affirming their reality and validity by integrating them into imagined human lives.

Yet whilst patients will likely find echoes of their own beliefs about time in these novels, drawing them in and gaining their attention, they may also find these beliefs challenged. The fluctuating emphases, and interplay of different ideas, constantly suggest alternative ways of interpreting experiences. Solzhenitsyn shows how narratives can expand moments, easing anxieties about life's brevity. Green also finds a way of interposing little infinities amongst the protracted periods of suffering cancer causes. Spiritual carers can use these novels to help patients regain control over their experiences of time. Pointing out the descriptive and imaginative resources the narratives contain, and the alternative outlooks tested within their fictional worlds, can give patients new ways of understanding the role time plays in their existence. Comments from participants in the focus groups and Fiction Library trial revealed, indeed, that reading and discussing *The Fault in Our Stars* can affirm a cancer patient's experiences of time, helping them to see that they are 'not the only one' struggling with their relationship to the temporal. Furthermore, participants' responses to *The Fault in Our Stars* showed how an appropriate fictional narrative can encourage patients to adopt a more active, constructive role in determining how their own time is described, organised and valued, embracing the 'idea of a long time [that] was completely different to the medical idea of a long time'. Furthermore, evidence from the trials demonstrates that a carefully selected fictional narrative can enable a cancer patient to identify and cherish the 'gifts' and 'seemingly contradictory' moments of joy and peace that can emerge amid a life disrupted or cut short by cancer.

Earlier in this chapter, I noted Lewis's concerns about cancer's propensity to expose the 'power of time to tease us' in a frantically paced modern world. There is an element of truth in his comments about Western society's 'fear of time's expanses', but the popularity of novels like *The Fault in Our Stars* suggests that this is not the whole story. Literature, films and television series which play with ideas of time-travel, relativity and infinity are a significant presence in popular culture.[119] Considered alongside other trends, like the increased interest in meditation and mindfulness,[120] and the rediscovery of the 'slow read',[121] there is evidence of a curiosity concerning the nature of time. The holes cancer treatment carves out in someone's life might give them the time to indulge this curiosity, and spiritual care could use fiction to support this voyage of discovery.

Chapter 4
CANCER, PARADOX AND *BREAKING BAD*

A cancer diagnosis forces a patient to search for meaning amidst pain, suffering, and a heightened awareness of their own mortality. In a society which is often accused of 'weakness' in its dealings with these subjects,[122] it is striking that millions of people have chosen to devote several hours to watching fictional character Walter White struggle with inoperable lung cancer in the television series *Breaking Bad*. This Netflix production is the foremost example of 'a TV landscape that's awash with death' says Craig Simpson: several recent series in which characters must 'come to terms with their own mortality'.[123] According to James Monaco the 'pervasive influence of television' means that shows like *Breaking Bad* are now 'part of our reality',[124] and its popularity suggests that people do not simply want to keep matters of death and suffering out of their everyday lives. I believe this influential, accessible modern medium could be used in spiritual care to enhance viewers' capacity for imaginative engagement with the theme of cancer and death.

The story of Walter White deals directly with this crucial aspect of cancer patients' experiences. Most patients are devastated and frustrated when they are first told they have cancer. They feel intense fear and must come to terms with what Grace Chu-Hui-Lin Chi terms a terrifying 'threat to hope'.[125] To be exposed to a disease which undermines expectations of security and comfort, and refocuses attention on sickness and survival, can be deeply unsettling, especially in a culture which seems to shy away from open discussion of suffering and death. Victor Frankl writes that a patient's search for meaning is often hampered by a 'lack of skill and language to deal with death' in modern society.[126] Many sociologists, psychiatrists, and cultural commentators have claimed that contemporary Western society is responsible for a dangerous 'denial of death'.[127] *Breaking Bad* conveys in dramatic form how, for a cancer patient trying to come to terms with the threat to hope and life posed by their disease, denial is not enough. The expansive scale of the series gives its viewers an opportunity for empathetic engagement with characters conditioned to see our human relationship to death as a battle which can never be won: a refusal to recognise the inevitable which leaves little room for a search for meaning.

As well as deepening its audience's understanding of the dangers of denial, *Breaking Bad* also uses the unique qualities of TV in unconventional approaches to cancer and mortality. Devices like shot selection, sequence and editing allow the camera to capture perspectives beyond the fear and confusion characters display, adding a depth of meaning to the drama. This invites viewers to consider the possibility of creative hope found amidst the chaos of cancer. In my own experience I found that *Breaking Bad* directly addresses this area of cancer patients' experiences, presenting audio-visual imagery which could transform viewers' attitudes towards the fragility and brevity of human life, giving cancer patients new perspectives on denial, fear, and mortality.[128]

Breaking Bad is a story about how a diagnosis of inoperable lung cancer leads an unassuming, mild-mannered chemistry teacher called Walter White (played by Bryan Cranston) to become a violent, notorious drug dealer. The first season shows Walt's (Walter's) diagnosis, and his decision to begin raising money to leave his family after his death by 'cooking' methamphetamine. He recruits petty criminal Jesse Pinkman – a former pupil – to help, and is immediately successful due to his specialist knowledge of the chemical processes involved. However, Walt's actions lead to him becoming increasingly estranged from his pregnant wife, Skyler, and son Walter Jr., who has cerebral palsy. Another source of jeopardy is Walt's brother-in-law, Hank, who works for the Drug Enforcement Agency (DEA) and is investigating the high-quality meth Walt has put onto the street. By the end of the first season, Walt's plan has started to spiral out of control, and he resorts to drastic means to achieve his goal.

Seasons 2 and 3 show Walt descending deeper into the corrupting world of drug-dealing. Still trying to preserve the crumbling remains of his family life, Walt starts to embrace immorality and violence. His attempts to be a stable, loving father-figure lose all credibility, and he even misses the birth of his new daughter to complete a lucrative drug deal. The tension is gradually ratcheted up, as Walt is sucked into a multi-million-pound drug trafficking network run by local businessman Gustavo Fring. Season 4 sees Walt trying to extricate himself from Fring's empire, which involves a deadly struggle between the two characters, culminating in Walt assassinating his boss using an improvised bomb. Meanwhile, Walt is still trying to balance this vicious conflict with his domestic life, even as Hank closes in on 'Heisenberg': the infamous criminal persona Walt has created for himself. During this time, Walt's cancer had gone into remission, granting him an unexpected reprieve, and buying him more time for his criminal enterprise. However, in season 5 the cancer returns in a more aggressive form, just as Hank finally realises that his own brother-in-law is the meth-cooking mastermind he has been chasing. Walt is forced into a lonely exile after one of his associates murders Hank, and his relationship with his family finally breaks down irreparably. But as his condition worsens, Walt opts to return for a final showdown, rather than succumb to his cancer alone. He is fatally wounded in this last blaze of bullets and violence, and is left by the camera to die, surrounded by bloodstained lab equipment.

Breaking Bad is seen by many as a landmark series that helped to drive a 'decisive shift' in television which began at the turn of the century.[129] Those trying to explain the widespread acclaim it has received often cite the 'cinematic look' of the series,[130] arguing this exemplifies the way in which television drama has 'reinvented itself' as a genre in recent years.[131] [132] [133]

Television critics have observed that from a 'storytelling perspective', television of this kind is 'more akin to novels than film'.[134] In the nineteenth century, reading serialised novels was a unifying experience, often done out-loud as a social, shared event. Consequently, they were often the main form of cultural and social expression.[135] There are clear similarities with the extent to which series like *Breaking Bad* have become what Robert Johnston calls 'arguably the most persuasive, powerful and ineluctable force of our time'.[136]

For spiritual carers seeking an influential, accessible

medium which can change our relationship to death and suffering, a series which tackles these themes in a manner which introduces new attitudes and possibilities into the midst of our lives could be a vital resource. Finding surprising, inventive perspectives on human mortality woven seamlessly into the rhythms of everyday life, even as these same rhythms are disrupted by the chaos of cancer, could be hugely helpful for many patients. Dramas like *Breaking Bad* can offer to help us to overcome the silences and hesitancy caused by the 'denial of death' in contemporary society.

Entire websites have been set up solely devoted to discussing the series,[137] as well as countless message boards.[138] Controversy surrounding ethical issues raised by its portrayal of cancer and family life received international press coverage.[139] The series has had as many as 1.2 million followers on Twitter,[140] and more than 11 million people were subscribed to its Facebook page.[141] [142]

The series uses its medium to capture three specific ways in which the medical and societal denial of death influences patients' experiences of cancer: the hostility, fear, and alienation that frequently characterise patients' reactions to diagnosis and treatment. Its portrayal of Walter White not only reflects and affirms these negative responses, but it also brings to light connections between the cancer ward, the public domain, and the family home, encouraging audiences to recognise how harmful attitudes of denial and evasion can be. *Breaking Bad* can feel like 'a show about us', argues Eric San Juan, not because it resonates with some subconscious yearning to manufacture illegal drugs, but because it plays on familiar, pervasive anxieties about death.[143] *Breaking Bad* distils and intensifies the narrative of the war against cancer, suggesting in drastic, dramatic form how this perspective might affect those involved.

In healthcare institutions, the medical treatment of cancer is often characterised as a violent assault against death and disease. As soon as they enter the clinic, says Edgar Jackson, 'the patient ill with cancer stands at the centre of an emotional battleground'.[144] Oncologists and nurses often employ battle terminology: the language of 'staying strong' and 'fighting' death.[145] Indeed, one patient, Nell Dunn, recalls being told that the clinicians would 'give her a real battering with platinum chemotherapy', as if this would bring comfort and reassurance.[146] Patients' bodies are caught in the crossfire, as treatment like chemotherapy involves using 'toxic' chemicals which work by indiscriminately 'damaging or interrupting cellular activity', an approach comparable, says Christie Watson, to 'taking a sledgehammer to a hazelnut'.[147] A 2019 BBC Horizon documentary about the need to 'talk about death' within the NHS describes how clinicians instinctively 'default to treatment A': the 'big treatment', when dealing with cancer.[148] There is a reluctance to entertain the idea of 'reconciliation with life and death', or a more constructive, optimistic acceptance of the inevitability of death.[149]

This medical characterisation of cancer treatment as a violent conflict clearly influences patients' understandings of their circumstances. Patients who cannot face the prospect of dying are quick to adopt the language of conflict as a way of expressing their desperate defiance. The testimony of one patient, Bob Cleland, who had a wife and two daughters, typifies this response: 'I was determined to beat whatever was wrong with me... for my family's sake I had to put a brave face on it'.[150] Machismo ideas of bravery and battling, inspired by the clinical campaign against cancer, harden patients' refusal to acknowledge the possibility of death. An attitude of angry, stubborn resistance proved the natural response for a father who felt he must 'beat' death. Moreover, because this language of conflict is so pervasive, and is used routinely by oncologists, nurses, friends and family members, it is difficult to avoid.

In the character of Walter White, we watch this violent opposition to cancer and death spill out into his life beyond the hospital. When Walt is given his diagnosis, his first reaction is to fight, and become more reckless.[151] The convictions driving this behaviour are gradually exposed over the course of the series, such as in a conversation between Walt and another cancer patient waiting for a CT scan. Dressed in medical gowns, and set against the backdrop of the cold, clinical hospital environment, Walt relates how he has concluded that his cancer must be fought: 'cancer is a death sentence, that's what they keep telling you'. He knows 'bad news' will come, but will not stop resisting: 'until then, who's in charge? Me!' [152] Until his 'death sentence' is fulfilled, Walt will continue to struggle against the inevitability of death, using chemistry and criminality to try to perform the role of the authoritative father-figure 'in charge' of his family's future. Walter's resistance elicited sympathetic responses from participants in the focus groups I ran, giving them a way of expressing personal frustrations and anxieties. This included the participant who explained that they could relate to Walt's desire to keep fighting because 'it's difficult for a man who was diagnosed with cancer... he wants to make sure he's got his family sorted financially'. Another participant described how Walt's desire to retain control resonated with them, explaining how a cancer diagnosis had conflicted with this instinctive desire: 'I'm a control freak, once I lost control and didn't know what was happening, my confidence went in other areas.'

In the focus groups there was also discussion of the

anger Walter displays – anger that several participants recognised as part of their personal reaction to cancer. One participant said that 'the anger that sometimes people [with cancer] show, I think this series [*Breaking Bad*] shows it's possible you might feel like that, and it's okay to be like that sometimes, because it's all part of the whole picture'. From this commentary, it seems clear that *Breaking Bad* is one example of a fictional narrative that could help cancer patients to access and speak about powerful emotions like anger which might otherwise remain unacknowledged. Yet watching Walter's narrative also led to reflection on the dangers of allowing oneself to be governed by the anger cancer causes. Collaboratively, those in the focus groups began to examine how the existential trauma of cancer can influence relationships, leading to hostility towards others. Several participants suggested that Walter was allowing an understandable sense of anger to shape his relationships. As one person put it, 'there can be such a lot of anger about what's happened to you, perhaps you take it out on the world?'. So there are fascinating parallels here between *Breaking Bad* and 'real' patient experiences.

Right to the bitter end, Walt continues to employ the language of war. In a particularly shocking scene, he tells his frightened, confused family, who have started to realise the full extent of his moral descent, that he will triumph over his cancer: 'I want to beat this thing... I'm back on chemo and I'm fighting like hell.' The audience sees this aggression in Walt's posture and expression, as he looms over his trembling wife and children. The medium combines the threatening physicality of Walt's body language with the distressing sounds of children's tears and screams, intensifying the impact of this furious tirade. Walt embodies fiery, passionate denial to the last. Such moments are ingenious because they hold together the relatable and repulsive.[153] Walt's defiant rhetoric captures a reaction to cancer that is both common and comprehensible in the context of modern society: a 'bravery' and fighting spirit many might see as laudable. Yet, in Walter White the superficially admirable collides with the brutally criminal, challenging the audience to reflect on the violent values of conflict and denial which influence patients and carers.

Breaking Bad also encourages cancer patients to consider how and why they might have chosen to deny death and disease. Walt exemplifies a form of 'calculative' reason that represents what Lisa Kadonaga calls a 'very modern, rational way of thinking'.[154] His personal philosophy is typical of a recognisable, relatable fixation with 'empirical science', and the 'goal of understanding and controlling a complex world'.[155] Because of this, the series presents an empathetic, nuanced understanding of why patients become complicit in the rationalising, controlling medical war on death. And this helps us understand how this perspective has become so influential.

Walt's reliance on 'calculative reason', and obsession with 'controlling a complex world', is exposed throughout the series. In an episode in season 3 entitled 'Fly', the discovery of a housefly in Walt's carefully maintained meth-lab environment results in an 'Ahab-like mission to kill it': a campaign against the offending contaminant which occupies the entire episode.[156] Walt's high-tech machinery is useless against this unexpected enemy, and the fruitless hunt becomes a metaphor for his war against another unwanted intrusion: death. Nothing in his scientific armoury can help in the fight against the fly, and the audience is given an entire episode to reflect on the limitations of Walter's stubborn, materialist worldview when it is confronted with the unpredictable and ungovernable forces of nature and mortality. His behaviour provides similar insight to the story of a real patient who continued the war against death by trying to annihilate all traces of dirt and germs in her home, in a desperate attempt to re-establish a sense of control. Having been treated in the 'physically and emotionally sterilised atmosphere of a hospital' she created an environment in her own home in which 'a germ couldn't live for thirty seconds', using chemical products to attack 'ghosts of the past', and continue the war against disease and death.[157] Like Walt, the patient had adopted the toxic scientific weapons of denial, but had learned nothing about accepting or living with death. The audience sees Walt unwittingly reveal these connections between the way medical practice approaches the problem of death, and smaller, everyday manifestations of the 'very modern' fixation with 'controlling a complex world'.

A more extreme, jarring instance of this insight comes through Walt and Jesse's treatment of the body of a drug dealer, whom they accidentally kill in the second episode of the series. To dispose of the evidence, Walt suggests they resort to 'chemical disincorporation': scientific jargon for dissolving the body in acid. Walt uses his scientific expertise to annihilate all traces of the man's death, whilst also avoiding direct discussion of the deed. Euphemistic references to 'the body situation' and 'the thing' betray Walt and Jesse's unwillingness to engage with the human dimension of their victim's death. Whilst they wipe up the gruesome physical remains from the 'disincorporation', a revealing sequence of flashbacks shows the audience a younger Walt in a classroom, explaining how science can account for '99.88804%' of the human body's composition, before concluding 'there's nothing but chemistry here'.

Clever editing links Walt's conviction that 'chemistry and matter is 'all of life'' to the murderous path his cancer diagnosis has taken him down.[158]

Underlying Walt's unacceptable, idiosyncratic criminality is a fear of death that elicits empathy, mirroring the 'panic' and 'hopelessness' cancer patients feel. The series recreates the unsettling surroundings of a cancer ward, revealing how this environment can incite and sustain these feelings, and translating them into a reaction which all viewers can comprehend.

Driving the preference for the aggressive treatment of cancer in the modern clinic is a sense of fear and confusion. Doctors and nurses often refer to hesitancy and unease surrounding the subject of death amongst their colleagues. Oncologist Mark Porter writes openly about this atmosphere: '[l]ike many of my colleagues I struggle to talk about prognosis when the outlook is bleak'.[159] Clinicians are thrust into an environment in which suffering and death are prominent, pressing concerns, without the emotional or spiritual literacy to talk directly and honestly about these human realities. Patients voice their frustration at the reticence they encounter when they raise these subjects: 'I need my doctor to discuss the possibility of death'.[160] Yet doctors told psychiatrist Elisabeth Kübler-Ross that 'many of us avoid any talk of death' because of 'the awful and unbearable feeling that there is nothing we can say or do'.[161]

When they are first diagnosed, a cancer patient is 'confronted with [their] finiteness in an abrupt and harrowing way'.[162] Patients are rarely prepared for this shock, and surveys show that the mere mention of cancer 'conjures visions of 'pain', 'fear', 'hopelessness' and 'inevitable death'.[163] The consequences of brushing mortality 'under the carpet' in contemporary life and the modern clinic is that patients instinctively respond to cancer with feelings of 'desperation and hopelessness' and the 'adoption of a fatalistic attitude'.[164] [165] Patients' stories often indicate that time in hospital undergoing cancer treatment exacerbates these fears about the loss of security and safety.[166]

Breaking Bad uses its medium to immerse the audience in this unsettling 'parallel universe' which would otherwise remain unknown to everyone except cancer patients, thus bridging the gap between Normality and the World of Cancer. In the first episode, we see Walt in an MRI scanner, shot from above and upside-down. The camera angle, Walt's bewildered expression, and the loud, mechanical noises emanating from the machine create a disorientating experience for the viewer, making it easy to share in Walt's anxiety. When Walt moves into the oncologist's office, the noise from the machine is carried over as an intrusion, ensuring the audience can only hear blurred, incomprehensible speech. Like Walt, the viewer cannot grasp or process the conversation, and the distorting mechanical sounds are only removed in time for us to hear 'Lung cancer. Inoperable... do you understand?'. Showing no evidence that he has understood this news, Walt can only comment on a mustard stain on the oncologist's tie that has drawn his attention, distracting from the devastating diagnosis that he has just received.[167]

The blurred speech, din, and unsettling atmosphere were evocative for many participants in the focus groups. These effects captured an emotional state that several of the patients involved in the groups recognised. As one participant put it: 'he lived in a panic mode – that's what I did!'. Others interpreted Walt's behaviour as a dramatic illustration of the difference between hearing and understanding a diagnosis, such as the participant who said Walt's dazed incomprehension reflected their immediate response to diagnosis: 'it's like: 'I've got this in an instant, but it's not permeated through me yet''. Describing a similar experience, a patient borrowed the visual metaphor of Walt's strange fascination with the oncologist's tie to explain how their reaction to diagnosis contrasted with their spouse's, saying: 'the whole thing seemed to hit her right there and then, whereas I'm still looking at this bit of mustard on a tie [i.e., not processing the news]'.

Evidently, the scene provided several participants with audio-visual tools that aided reflection and enriched their storytelling. This was also apparent when a patient likened Walt's behaviour during the scan and meeting to meditation, suggesting the sound and sights 'become something different to focus on... you've got the beat [of the MRI machine] to focus on then you've got the mustard spot to focus on'. Identifying with Walt, they said 'it's how you deal with things sometimes – it's a bit like meditation, allowing your brain to formulate [ideas] when things are too emotional'.

These comments highlight how the scene gives the audience privileged access to the post-diagnosis 'daze' that real patients describe: the feeling that they had slipped into a 'dark, lonely' nightmare in which meaningful communication becomes impossible. Indeed, one participant in the focus groups responded to this scene by describing how it captured their feelings following diagnosis: 'I think it portrayed the emotion of that [learning a diagnosis], it was really well done'. In fact, the discussion of this scene in the focus groups led several participants to speak about their 'petrifying' or 'extremely stressful' experiences of undergoing an MRI scan. Walt embodies the solitude of the lone individual trapped in the bleak murkiness of the 'World of Cancer', reminiscent of the real patient whose experience of the MRI was like being in a 'plastic coffin'.[168]

Furthermore, this commentary led some of the healthcare professionals involved in the focus groups to consider how patients' need for meditation or distraction, buying time to process shocking news, could be accommodated. Having listened to the comments this scene elicited from patients, they recognised the importance of making allowances for coping mechanisms that may seem strange or irrational. For instance, a healthcare professional suggested that the oncologist could have participated in Walt's 'meditation', giving him space to come to terms with his prognosis by supporting his deflection strategy: 'you kind of thought [the oncologist] could have said, 'I had a burger for lunch' or something [to explain the mustard stain], but there was just no reaction'. Collaboratively, through discussions of the clip, patients and providers appeared to be moving towards a clearer understanding of why this encounter felt unsatisfactory, whilst also testing out alternative approaches to these interactions. One caregiver expressed this perfectly when they said that the clip had encouraged them to consider how to 'show a bit of humanness' when interacting with patients, searching for 'some kind of connection' with the people they were treating.[169]

As we see Walt 'made aware of his own embodied existence as a finite being' in the dominant 'culture of widespread death anxiety' within healthcare institutions, we better understand the way cancer throws this tension into sharp relief.[170]

At the heart of a new and better way of understanding and living with cancer is the idea of paradox – that something good and positive can emerge from the awfulness of facing a deadly illness.

CANCER, PARADOX AND *BREAKING BAD*

In cancer care meaning must be, as Brian Maclaren argues, 'sought or constructed in the midst of pain and tears'.[171] Simply telling patients to find meaning by ignoring or overcoming feelings of anger, fear and loneliness, rather than recognising them as natural, relatable responses, will not work. However, it is also clear from patient experiences, and the way these are depicted in Walter White's story, that as Mick Brandon puts it 'to allow cancer to take the lead will always leave us bankrupt': spiritually 'impoverished' and trapped in meaninglessness.[172] *Breaking Bad* suggests how hope and consolation can be reached 'because of', not 'in spite of' patients' acceptance of death and sickness.[173] Arthur Koestler argued that modern 'technological man' has 'forgotten that the awareness of our own mortality can render our lives more valuable, more precious'.[174] Whilst Walter White encapsulates the spiritual limitations of the 'technological man', the aesthetics, imagery and depth of meaning in *Breaking Bad* suggest other approaches to mortality, which could help patients to seek out more optimistic, 'precious' meanings.

A show like *Breaking Bad* can introduce patients to paradoxical possibilities of life, hope and strength found amidst death and disease. Carers can use *Breaking Bad* to introduce patients to the notion of positive paradox, giving them the 'renewed skill set for facing their own mortality' that 'people today require'.[175]

An elderly woman in a cancer ward trying to express her experience of hospital drew a picture of her surroundings. Above the image of the ward, she wrote the words 'faith', 'hope' and 'care', but below it she put 'shock', 'wilderness' and 'frightening'.[176] Her drawing became a constructive collection of contradictory reactions: a thoughtful rendering of what John Swinton calls 'creative resignation', which acknowledged fear and shock whilst preserving faith and hope.[177] [178] Another patient, trying to come to terms with the loss of her hair to chemotherapy, describes how she 'felt like a fraud' wearing a wig, as it seemed she was 'somehow denying [her] illness'. Reconciling herself to this loss allowed her to feel purposeful again and 'enriched her life'.[179] Directly confronting her new appearance, she did not see a *memento mori* but found meaning by openly displaying the signs of her illness.

Rosemary Gordon argues that there are several similarities between 'those who would die well and those who would create well', contending that both death and creation require us to 'hear doubt and chaos and not-knowing, without excessive panic'.[180] Calm, confident acceptance of the chaos of cancer can foster the kind of creativity which flows out from darkness, painting positive paradoxes in the colours of despair, and communicating hope through the 'language of suffering'. The way these patients work with the 'apparently paradoxical association of feelings' like 'inspiration and fear' reveals a crucial alternative to the denial of death.[181]

On one level, Walter White embodies creativity in the face of death. His decision to turn his scientific skills to cooking meth of the highest quality shows admirable ingenuity and imagination. He rejects the 'Cancer Man' identity – the passive, anxious 'image of a cancer patient' – and chooses 'the more fearsome "Heisenberg" persona instead', giving his life a new meaning and direction.[182] The creative, inspirational aspects of his response to cancer are captured in Jesse's stunned appraisal of the first batch of drugs Walt produces: 'You're a goddamn artist ... This is art'. A 'lyrical cook sequence' using 'flashy editing and cool music', combined with the 'slick compression of time and effort' has already portrayed this as a stylish, impressive process, letting the audience share in Jesse's wonder at Walt's technical prowess.[183] The manipulation of sound, sequence and shot makes it difficult not to see Walt in this moment as what James Parker describes as a 'Mozart in the land of meth': a genius 'touched with artistic fire'.[184] When Gordon refers to the paradoxical associations between 'good and peaceful dying' and 'creative work', this seems to be relevant to what Walt has achieved. Like the patients who were able to find reasons for faith and hope in the depths of despair, Walt often appears to be a model of 'creative resignation'.[185] Indeed, a fellow chemist with whom Walt cooks in the third season draws attention to Walt's capacity for creativity by comparing him to Walt Whitman, his 'other favourite W. W.' and a 'poet' with the vision to 'look up and out of the world'. [186]

The ingenuity of Walt's response to cancer is also embodied in his hair. In a significant scene in season 1, the viewer watches Walt, who has begun to notice the side-effects of chemotherapy, playing with his thinning hair in the mirror, before picking up a razor. The next shot, before we see Walt's new haircut, shows the stunned reactions of Skyler and Walter Jr. as Walt enters the room. He has shaved his head entirely, embracing his changing appearance, and the audience first witnesses this reflected in the stunned faces of his family, and his son's delight and pride: 'Badass, dad!'.[187]

Here, the manipulation of shot and sequence means we first 'see' Walt's baldness through the reactions of Walt's astonished family members, whose assumptions about living with cancer are suddenly disrupted. Walt's chaotic progress towards infamy and evil includes says Todd DuBose moments of liberating 'freedom' and 'artistry', mixed into the 'maelstrom of gale-force-winded values in flux'.[188] Like the patient who 'enriched' her life by accepting hair loss and openly acknowledging her disease and its treatment, Walt seems momentarily to epitomise courageous, honest reconciliation with cancer. In a show which often 'suspends... our narratives of common sense', argues Pamela Brown and 'pushes them in unexpected directions',[189] Walt's spontaneous shaving appears to model this paradoxical use of loss as an opportunity for re-creation.

Although patients' initial reactions to a cancer diagnosis are frequently characterised by fear, anger and denial, several patients also describe gradually reaching a realisation that 'cancer teaches you to live' and can be the 'beginning of a new life path'.[190] There are elements of Walt's response to his diagnosis which hint at this paradox, challenging the idea that life and death are antithetical, and opening up the notion of death as a source of 'new life' for viewers to explore.[191]

Walt's dealings with cancer and death begin and end with him discussing life, framing his entire story as an examination of life and death held in balance. When Jesse asks, in the first episode, if Walt is 'crazy or depressed', and questions why he would turn to a life of crime, Walt declares that he is alive and alert: 'I am awake ... we start tomorrow'. Returning to this theme in the final episode of the series, Walt explains his outrageous, vicious behaviour by saying 'I did it for me... I was alive'. In all the wrong ways, Walt has been searching for meaningful life. He 'wakes up and recognises that his life is transient' says Stephen Glass,[192] then tries to respond with direct, decisive action. Like those patients who began to 'look forward' and 'found a new path in life' because of their cancer, Walt starts searching for a new direction. And because this gives the audience a new awareness of this paradox, this is 'a new 'plan of life' that may contain elements of truth despite its illegality.[193]

One excellent example of the challenge *Breaking Bad* presents to conventional ideas about this theme is the family 'intervention' scene in season 1, episode 5. Skyler has assembled the family, including Marie and Hank, in a bid to persuade Walt to undergo chemotherapy, something he has resisted up to this point. Like the clinicians who instinctively resort to 'big treatment', Skyler is convinced that using toxic chemicals to attack Walt's cancer is the only viable course of action. She insists it is in his 'best interests', telling Walt 'you need the treatment, and nothing can stop you from getting it'. Emboldened by his mother's passion, Walter Jr. mocks his father for being 'scared of a little chemotherapy', but Walt's riposte to his loved ones raises a very different possibility. He condemns the medical culture that sees 'doctors talking about surviving as if it's the only thing that matters', and often leaves patients 'artificially alive' and 'just marking time'. Those real patients who found meaning though facing up to mortality, and holding life and death in balance, would share Walt's belief that living well is not solely about deferring death.[194]

A Maggie's psychologist participating in the Fiction Library trial specifically identified *Breaking Bad* as an artwork that raised the same questions of quantity and quality of life that many visitors to the Maggie's centre were grappling with. In their feedback, the psychologist described how they felt the series raised relevant, important themes for the people they cared for:

'When thinking about *Breaking Bad*, I can see how people begin to think about their legacy and what they can do for those that are left behind before they die. It is an interesting conversation regarding prolonging life vs quality of life. Working in the [Maggie's] centre this topic has come up in regards to the importance of people having a voice and being able to say "enough is enough" in regards to treatment. People may prolong their life, but if it is not a quality life, I think there needs to be respect for deciding to stop or not take up treatment.'

The discovery that *Breaking Bad* can be used to open up this increasingly important area of patients' experiences is highly significant. The psychologist's remarks suggested that *Breaking Bad* can reveal why cancer patients will begin to 'think about their legacy' or 'those that are left behind', highlighting the potential relevance of Walt's narrative for those Maggie's cares for. Watching and discussing *Breaking Bad* could afford a way into the sensitive 'conversation' about quality and quantity of life that many patients feel that they need to have, as the psychologist's response to the series implied.

Furthermore, evidence from the focus groups clearly showed me that the intervention scene could indeed initiate constructive conversations about this vital subject. One person responded to the intervention scene by speaking about a friend who was determined to continue caring for his wife after he was diagnosed with cancer. They related how the friend 'wouldn't have the chemo, because he knew he'd have the reaction to the chemo, and he wasn't going to be there for his wife. So, he cut his life short by not having any treatment'. Walt's resistance to treatment drew out this story, as it seemed to touch on precisely the same concerns that motivated Walt. Another participant expressed their approval of Walter's decision, saying, 'I know there are people who, quite rightly, found that they decided not to have chemotherapy'. As they explained, their endorsement of this choice was due to personal experiences of treatment, as they said that 'I had such a bad time that I'd never go through chemo again'. These participants, and many others, found their compelling reasons for resisting treatment captured in Walter's speech to his family.

Yet there were also examples of the scene provoking the opposite reaction, moving people to speak about their positive experiences of treatment. One participant told the group about their daughter, who continued to play an active role in family life whilst undergoing chemotherapy. They explained that their daughter had 'participated in our lives a lot during that time' noting that 'it's not been a case of giving up and lying down in bed all day'. This challenge to Walter's portrayal of life during treatment was echoed by another person who objected to the way their doctors had characterised treatment. They asked, 'why do they have to tell you all the bad things that are going to happen?', adding that 'I had radiotherapy, I was told I would be very tired, but I wasn't, it was fine'. These comments indicate that Walter's distrust of treatment can also draw out different stories and experiences. The scene thus provided the basis for rich, nuanced conversations in the groups – conversations that seemed to do justice to the complexity of the issues raised.

So I believe *Breaking Bad* could be used to help people to explore these issues, privately or in groups. And one participant in the groups had a suggestion for how this might work best in practice. Noting that it engaged with the question of 'quality vs quantity of life' that many patients confront, the participant argued that it would be wise to pair *Breaking Bad* with a fictional narrative presenting a more positive perspective on cancer treatment. In their words, 'to have something to counter it would be really, really helpful'. The balance between extending life and preserving its quality is difficult to find and will vary for each individual. Yet current cancer care provision does not usually support a patient's search for this balance. As these discussions revealed, integrating fictional explorations of this issue into their spiritual care could both initiate and enrich this search.

At certain points, *Breaking Bad* uses its medium to guide audience attention towards the paths Walter White did not take: the help and love he chose to ignore, and the paradox that he weakened his position by refusing to accept support. Cancer patients frequently experience isolation and what's been called 'existential aloneness'.[195] They can feel as if they have become as Todd Dubose puts it the dreaded 'image of a cancer patient': a '*memento mori*' or reminder of our mortality in a society desperate to deny death's reality.[196] The language of 'fighting' death can also push patients towards loneliness and isolation. John Swinton observes that an ideal of self-sufficiency is directly connected with the metaphors of fighting disease, which 'work well in an individualistic society' in which we are encouraged to be 'autonomous heroes'.[197] As cancer support specialist Pamela Brown observes, patients are often conditioned to believe 'that it's a strength to be independent, to not ask for help'.[198] The extent to which Walt aspires to an ideal of 'strength' and independence is exposed in the moments of insulating, indulgent egotism in which he distances himself from his family, such as when he proclaims in a grandiose, melodramatic speech: 'I have lived under the threat of death for a year now, and because of that I've made choices ... I alone should suffer the consequences'. Leaving loved ones behind, Walt makes clear his intention to face cancer alone. He has clearly come to regard himself as an 'autonomous hero' who must fight cancer without support. However, there is also a very different perspective on cancer and human relationships which often emerges in patient testimonies. Many patients say that their experience of cancer has resulted in 'a fresh realisation that we are interdependent' – a renewed appreciation of the strength and spiritual support that can be gained through reliance on those around us.[199]

Ironically, it is Walter White's failure to embrace this paradox which makes Breaking Bad an excellent resource for encouraging patients to consider the importance of dependence on others. Sometimes culture can be most effective by showing the consequences of a path not taken, of not behaving in a particular way. There is a tradition within Christian art of imagery which portrays evil in the form of a 'silhouette of goodness': a 'negative image' of virtue in which sin becomes an absence that points towards a better path not chosen.[200] Breaking Bad uses its narrative and aesthetics in an analogous way, depicting Walt's assertions of independence, and rejection of help and sympathy, as a revealing 'silhouette' of alternative decisions he could have made, and of the strength he would have gained by submitting to dependence.

Patient testimonies stress the importance of such decisions. Journalist Victoria Derbyshire relates how 'experiencing cancer showed [her] that ninety-nine percent of people are kind'. She writes that she was initially shocked by having to 'confront the possibility of life being taken from [her]', but that she has now reached a point where she feels 'grateful... every single day', thanks to the 'compassionate words of wonderful strangers'[201] Paradoxically, the prospect of losing her life created a situation in which she discovered gratitude, mutuality and resilience. Sara Liyanage also describes how she found that the 'parallel universe' of life with cancer 'wasn't as lonely as [she] had first thought'. Despite seeing her diagnosis as the destruction of 'comfort' and end of 'Normality', she came to understand that 'you aren't as alone as you think', and found new sources of 'warmth, love and support' through fellow sufferers.[202] Liyanage's story suggests that something which might appear to transform a person into a disquieting sign of death cut off from community and friendship, can in fact lead a patient towards meaningful, affirming relationships, and a deeper appreciation of the importance of shared experience.

This paradox can also hold true in the context of family life. One patient reached the conclusion that 'cancer is a life changing experience', not because it forced him to fear for his life but because of the way it changed his relationships: 'my whole family is closer than we've ever been'. The way those around this patient responded to his diagnosis revealed 'a love so powerful that it began a healing process that forever changed [him].'[203] Counterintuitively, cancer prompted reconciliation and a strengthening of bonds: a restoring and strengthening with clear spiritual significance. For a father facing a potentially fatal cancer, this revelation came when he decided to be 'open', and 'talked to both [his] children about death'. Though he 'could not stop crying', he later recognised that discussing death with his family had been a crucial stage in his spiritual recovery: 'I think I needed that low moment in a strange way'.[204] Admitting to his fear of death, rather than denying its possibility, produced reassurance and courage – a new high attained by accepting and expressing the 'low'.

The capacity for *Breaking Bad* to encourage cancer patients to embrace dependence was evident from the responses in my focus groups to Walter's decision to receive his cancer diagnosis alone. Seeing Walter, disorientated and dazed, failing to process what the oncologist is telling him, several participants chose to speak about the importance of involving other people in hospital appointments and consultations. Having watched the scene in which Walter attends an MRI scan then receives his cancer diagnosis alone, one participant suggested that Walter should have brought another person to the consultation: 'I think it would have been better for him to have somebody with him. But that's your choice'.[205]

Interrogating Walter's choices led them to consider and propose an alternative course of action. This sentiment was repeated many times in each of the groups where *Breaking Bad* was discussed, as participants spoke about the necessity of bringing other people to appointments and involving friends and family in their treatment.

In a revealing scene towards the end of the fourth season of *Breaking Bad*, Walter Jr. finds his father cut, bruised and fragile, following an altercation with his drug-dealing associates. In a 'low moment' of weakness, Walt suddenly opens up to his son about his own experience of seeing his father in hospital dying of Huntington's disease. The unexpected, poignant qualities of this image of a weeping, battered cancer patient highlight what Walt has been missing up to this point: the new meaning which can come through submitting to weakness and reliance. When Walt tries to reinstate the façade of the strong, solitary cancer-warrior the next day, his son's reaction serves to reinforce this message: 'at least last night you were real'. When the real father reached his tearful 'low moment', sharing the burden of his fragility with his family, it led to hopeful spiritual resurgence, yet Walt treats his own slip into honesty as a display of vulnerability he does not want to repeat.[206] Walt's uncharacteristic moment of truthful humanity demonstrates how cinematic television can give audiences spiritually illuminating hints of 'wholeness': tantalising, fleeting visions of how Walt could have allowed healing love and support to transform his experience of cancer.[207]

Breaking Bad consistently points to this paradoxical possibility of 'wholeness' amidst the fractured chaos of cancer. In the final season, Walt celebrates his birthday with his family by giving a speech thanking his loved ones for their support: 'I did not want to get any treatment, I think I was too angry, too scared... but you guys got me through it'. Superficially, Walt's words reflect the experiences of patients whose struggles with cancer brought them closer to their families, deepening their spiritual resources. However, the viewer sees this deceitful display of hollow gratitude set against a backdrop of Skyler, distraught and despairing after learning about Walt's misdeeds, slowly walking into their family pool in an attempt to drown herself. The effect of placing these two figures in a single shot is a shockingly discordant scene, with Walt oblivious to the way his wife's tragic behaviour is exposing the cynicism of his speech, even as he delivers it. Walt's monologue ends up showing us how things might have been – how his family and friends could have given him the practical and spiritual support he needed to endure his treatment.

This kind of insight has very deep cultural roots going back a lot further than the modern era of TV shows. The vision of hell Dante Alighieri creates in his *Commedia* is a revealing example of this creative, hopeful use of the vacuity of immorality. It is full of lonely, isolated individuals who chose to 'abandon themselves to the emptiness of evil' and submit to 'dullness and death'.[208] Yet Robin Kirkpatrick points out that Dante describes his 'authorial task' within the *Inferno* as a struggle to write of 'the good I found there'

(*Inferno* I:7-8): to create a narrative with the 'moral and intellectual purpose' of using the bitterness of sin and death to evoke imaginative images of goodness.[209] In Dante's poetry the 'emptiness of evil' serves as a 'negative image' of a possible good,[210] just as the hellish existence Walt has trapped himself in is portrayed as a life that points to the better choices he did not make.[211]

The medium through which this jarring mismatch is presented also adds further layers of irony and tension to the shot. Monaco points out that 'it is in our personal lives, in our families, that the power of television has its most immediate effect'.[212] Series like *Breaking Bad* are usually watched with close friends or family, providing one of the commonest points of discussion among people today[213] and generating 'water-cooler' moments which make us want to share our views and responses.[214] In this context, witnessing the total collapse of familial bonds laid out in such a disturbing manner will inevitably focus the minds of those watching on the need to preserve trust and communication. The 'negative images' the series presents invite them to discuss with their own loved ones how things could have been handled differently, and Walt's cancer might have brought his family closer, leading to important conversations about how hope and consolation could be co-created by cancer patients and their families.

The potential value of this was illustrated in the feedback provided by a participant in the Fiction Library trial I established. Whilst processing the impact of a cancer diagnosis, the participant watched *Breaking Bad* having read in the Fiction Library guide about how the series could help them to explore themes of denial and dependence:

When I did watch episode 1 of *Breaking Bad*, I reflected on my relationship with my family since the diagnosis and immediately set about changing it. I thought I had been open with them but reading the comments [in the Fiction Library guide] about Walter's behaviour, I realised that I had tried to protect them and in doing so, was denying myself some much-needed support and them the opportunity of supporting me, which they were seeking and might even need as part of their process of coming to terms with the life-threatening illness of their daughter and sister. I wrote them an eight-page letter letting myself speak freely about how I felt about my situation to give them an idea of what it was like to be me. Following that, I had a much more meaningful exchange with my sister and mother.

Watching *Breaking Bad* in conjunction with reading the Fiction Library guide led this participant to a vital realisation. A narrative about the breakdown of family relationships provoked an important process of reflection, resulting in the participant seeking out more meaningful contact and mutual support. When they related to Walter's behaviour, the guide invited them to consider how the instinct to protect family members from the truth could have damaging consequences. The participant's response illustrated how, just as Dante's poetic forms were able to 'derive "good" even from the confusions of hell',[215] the desolate, destructive qualities of Walt's misdeeds serve a 'moral and intellectual purpose' by conjuring visions of their opposites. In this respect, *Breaking Bad* shows how the 'power of television' can be used as a platform through which viewers explore together alternative, paradoxical perspectives on cancer and death, and rethink assumptions about the need for patients to fear and fight death on their own.

Conclusion

One of the most valuable things *Breaking Bad* offers its audience is the opportunity to spend several hours watching somebody get life with cancer catastrophically wrong. In contemporary society, cancer often reaches the public's attention through stories about 'inspirations' and 'cancer heroes': extraordinary individuals who have run marathons, climbed mountains, or raised vast sums of money for charity.[216] Whilst impressive and admirable, the ideal of the patient who has 'beaten' cancer by achieving remarkable feats does little to address the fears about death and dying most ordinary patients contend with. In contrast, *Breaking Bad* is a notable example of an artwork willing to explore the human frailties that cancer exposes. The series provides the 'negative images' and 'silhouettes' which society does not offer, and which give the viewer the freedom to imagine what they would do instead, and how they would respond to cancer differently, rather than asking them to measure up against a daunting, unattainable ideal. Walt's story probes medical, societal and individual shortcomings, laying bare the problem death poses in our lives with an uncompromising candour that can be hard to find elsewhere.

What makes the series such a promising resource for spiritual care is the way in which it balances this brutal honesty with an awareness of how, as Ernest Becker says, 'the prospect of death ... wonderfully concentrates the mind',[217] introducing audiences to the paradoxical idea that something which threatens to take you out of the world can bring you more deeply into it. Cancer patients describe the 'pain' and 'hopelessness' their condition causes, and the terror death holds for them. Yet their testimonies also often point to this paradox, describing feelings of relief and renewal when death becomes closer and more familiar. *Breaking Bad* holds these two kinds of responses together in the same space. My own research shows cancer patients finding their feelings of fear, anger, and denial captured by the aesthetics, characterisation, and narrative of *Breaking Bad*, yet also being moved by the series to contemplate alternative perspectives on cancer and mortality.[218][219]

A counter-cultural movement encouraging people to discuss death and dying directly and openly is gradually gaining traction, and television documentaries,[220] podcasts,[221] children's animated films, [222] and even outlets in shopping centres such as the 'Departure Lounge' in Lewisham[223] are all playing a part in this drive to overcome our collective denial. *Breaking Bad* is a crucial testament to this broader trend, in which alternative attitudes towards our unavoidable end are being sought out and investigated. The imaginative space the series creates is one in which unorthodox ideas of creative resignation become viable possibilities, and viewers can rediscover the kind of spiritual optimism which finds glimmers of light in the darkness of death.

Chapter 5
THE BUCKET LIST: LEVITY, LAUGHTER AND LIVING WITH CANCER

In an enigmatic scene towards the end of Hollywood 'cancer comedy' *The Bucket List*, Cole, played by Jack Nicholson, is reflecting on the journey he has made with his friend Carter (Morgan Freeman).[224] As two terminal cancer patients, Cole and Carter decided to use their remaining life to tick off items on an extravagant 'bucket list', leading to a series of adventures full of levity and laughter. As he tries to understand the significance of these adventures, Cole turns to his colleagues in a meeting and asks: 'have you ever read the *Divine Comedy*?' [225] Seeking a means of expressing the transformative impact of fun and frivolity on his life with cancer, Cole chooses the example of a theological, 'Divine' comedy. I'm really interested in this kind of unexpected connection, and in this chapter I use *The Bucket List*, an odd-couple cancer comedy that drew large audiences[226] as an example of how filmic fun could enrich the spiritual care of cancer patients.

A failure to take comedy seriously is a feature of many different disciplines, including those tasked with addressing the human problems of death and disease.[227]

Both oncologists and patients have identified humour as a means of 'spiritual coping' that can improve mental and physical wellbeing, but carers are still searching for what are called 'effective humorous interventions'. At the moment a chasm exists between what cancer patients need and desire regarding humour, and the reality of what their care provides.[228][229] Responses to *The Bucket List* in focus groups I ran showed the film bringing relief, inspiring defiance, changing patient's perspectives on humour, and even prompting patients to re-evaluate their life goals.

The Bucket List is firmly focused on entertaining audiences by generating laughter and enjoyment. It sits within a category of films that is frequently accused of being 'vulgar', dismissed by scholars as 'mindless' entertainment.[230] Certain critical responses to *The Bucket List* characterised it as a 'popcorn picture about death',[231] with critics treating the film as a deplorable demonstration that 'Hollywood never found a cancer ward it couldn't spiff up' or 'a death sentence that didn't have emotional uplift'.[232] Whilst some responded favourably to this 'emotional uplift' other critics were dismissive of what they saw as 'putatively heart-warming stuff' that was ultimately 'lazy and condescending'.[233] There's even an implicit sense in a few reviews that those who enjoyed *The Bucket List* and its portrayal of 'cancer that is nothing like cancer' should feel ashamed,[234] with one reviewer suggesting that if you are won over by the film's 'cheerful defiance' it is important 'not to let your friends know'.[235] The underlying assumption of critics appears to have been that mixing illness and irreverence constituted a 'lazy' and 'disturbing' trivialisation of this dangerous disease.

However one need not look beyond recent examples like *The Greatest Showman* to realise that films that do best at the box office are rarely the critics' favourites so the reasons why millions of people choose to watch successful films like *The Bucket List* are rarely given detailed consideration.[236]

I believe comedy films like *The Bucket List* allow viewers to explore different ways of harnessing the power of comedy to change a life affected by cancer. They demonstrate how artworks can give viewers a means of vicariously experiencing different forms of comic response to cancer, testing out how humour might add to their own search for meaning. [237] The globe-trotting exploits of two dying men trying to cram fun and laughter into their final months offers audiences this opportunity. Furthermore, the increasing popularity of 'cancer comedy' as an 'emerging trend' in popular culture implies there is an appetite for accessible, entertaining narratives that allow people to explore ways of combining cancer and humour.[238]

Films which allow us to reflect on different uses of humour played out within imagined experiences of cancer also provide a space in which the limitations and power of laughter in this context can be tested out, at a safe distance from real life. Combining humour with serious illness requires sensitivity and an ability to adapt to individual preferences and unique circumstances,[239] so a medium which facilitates this encounter with the positive and negative dimensions of cancer comedy can be vitally important. Indeed, director Rob Reiner explains that his aim in creating *The Bucket List* was to 'present a very serious subject like [cancer] but also to inject humour, because if we're going to reflect the life experience it's sad and it's funny'.[240] He intended the film to entertain, yet in doing so to reflect and engage with real 'life experience'.

Using *The Bucket List* as an illustration, I will explain how Hollywood-style entertainment can be used to move from the finding that 'humour can be an effective intervention that impacts the health and wellbeing of patients with cancer' to a practicable care strategy.[241] Placing characters willing to poke fun at everything into situations all cancer patients will recognise leads to a playful, relatable hunt for the laughter which can be extracted from life with cancer. This is what this 'cancer comedy' offers: strategies for putting cancer, suffering and death into perspective using levity and laughter, which patients may find can be 'transferred' into their own lives. The relationship between Cole and Carter that is at the heart of *The Bucket List*, reveals how comedy can carry candour, denial or hopeful defiance with it when it is aimed at cancer.

So what exactly is the potential value of humour in this kind of situation? I've explored the academic debate about this among theologians and others in my doctoral work. What I believe is that theology helps us discover is that humour can really help people somehow see differently and rise above the situation they find themselves in. Hugo Rahner observes that 'fun, irony and humour' sometimes 'seem to get more easily – because more playfully – down to the truth'.[242] Ironic, dark or grotesque humour often 'employs distortion paradoxically as an instrument of truth', revealing the root of things by disturbing our preconceptions.[243] Humour's relationship to the truth is also sometimes characterised by its propensity for getting at those things which defy conventional logic and ordinary speech. Philosopher Slavoj Žižek suggests that because 'the stuff of comedy is things which elude our grasp', then 'laughter is one way of coping with the incomprehensible'.[244] Consequently, the comic hero can capture something of what it means to be a human beset by chaos and confusion, and do so with sympathy and honesty. Nathan Scott describes the clown as an 'utterly human' figure who 'somehow manages to redeem the human image' despite facing confusion and tragedy.[245] The downtrodden comic contending with the absurd, inexpressible qualities of life can still – against all the odds – present a faithful, hopeful image of what it means to be a person surrounded by 'things which elude our grasp'.

Playfulness and folly are also often discussed by theologians defending the religious significance of comedy. For instance, Conrad Hyers argues that comedy is spiritually vital because it can remind us of our 'intrinsic freedom and flexibility', by encouraging us to play around with possibilities and boundaries.[246] Because of this, ludic comedy can take the shape of a 'fantastic protest against the limitations of worldly existence'.[247] This belief also seems to lie behind Hugo Rahner's theology of play, in which the Christian *homo ludens* – 'man of play' – is a 'saint' who performs 'a children's game before God' from which 'every vestige of the tragic has completely disappeared'.[248] He asserts that a saint, far from being a figure associated exclusively with sobriety, can offer spiritual insight by playing a 'children's game' and delighting in disregarding the 'limitations of worldly existence'.

The imagery of levity as flight – light-heartedness as an escape from the gravity of weighty anxieties – is another theological account of the relationship between comedy and spirituality that I draw on.[249] This notion of 'godlike' ascendancy also lies behind artistic metaphors exploiting the association of levity with weightlessness and flight, such as in Dante Alighieri's *Commedia*, where humour and joy pull the protagonists towards the spiritual riches of Paradise and out of the density of despair.[250] Gavin Hopps highlights the 'religious allegory that is founded on the dual meaning of *levitas*', used in the *Commedia* to capture the significance of Dante's pilgrim's climb to the 'physical and spiritual "levity"' of paradise. Levity lets the believer fly towards the heavens, looking back with 'godlike' disdain on worldly burdens.

The Bucket List allows audiences to explore the various forms of relief and respite humour can bring to cancer patients. Nurses working in cancer wards quickly realise that humour is a crucial 'coping tool' that can reduce stress and aid relaxation.[251] The moments when characters in *The Bucket List* use comedy to escape from the grim reality of cancer can deepen our understanding of this important process. Paul Kalanithi writes that he learned about the therapeutic power of humour by watching his father – a clinician – use jokes to build trust and 'easy human connections' with patients. [252] Similarly, spending time in a cancer ward led nurse Christine Watson to the realisation that a smile or 'hearty gut-laugh' could cut through the 'horror of life' bringing patients respite.[253]

The Bucket List brings banter and slapstick comedy into a cancer ward, using the relationship between Cole and Carter to explore how humour can reassure or distract patients. As soon as Cole joins Carter on the ward, his antics transform the atmosphere. Falling out of his hospital bed in farcical style, he elicits a smile from his new ward companion. As the film's portrayal of time spent on a cancer ward develops, the relief that humour and fun bring is repeatedly emphasised. A shot of Cole, lying in his bed, feverish in his discomfort as the effects of chemotherapy set in, cuts straight to Cole and Carter, laughing and playing cards whilst bathed in sunlight.[254] The spiritual value of comic relief is further underlined through Cole's immediate response to his terminal cancer diagnosis. After a brief silence in the wake of hearing this devastating news, Carter does not ask Cole for his thoughts on the prognosis but suggests a game of cards. Cole's jovial reply – 'thought you'd never ask' – shows that the offer of a game has met his pressing need for play and distraction.[255] The audience experiences first-hand the respite moments of humour can afford, lightening the mood and buying patients time for processing shocking news.[256]

Oncologist Mark Porter explains that whilst working with cancer patients it is 'O.K. to laugh' as 'at the right moment humour can be a wonderful thing'.[257] Watching scenes in *The Bucket List* which blend tragedy and comic relief gives those watching an insight into why and when humour can be 'wonderful': a tool for exploring when the 'right moment' could be. This type of imaginative investigation is vital because it deepens viewers' understanding of the extent to which the power of humour is bound up in the context of individual patients and personal preferences. When Carter decides to join Cole in the pursuit of joy and adventure abroad, instead of remaining with his family and continuing treatment, his wife struggles to accept his decision. We see her explaining her concerns to Cole on the phone, begging him to persuade her husband to return as she can't bear to 'lose' him. The film cuts from this conversation to Carter luxuriating in Cole's ostentatious bathroom, soaking in a spacious marble bathtub lined with golden trim. And the scene immediately following this shows Cole and Carter on safari in Africa, singing and laughing as they enjoy their latest exotic jaunt. The tension this sequence creates – between the concern and confusion of Carter's wife, and his relaxation and laughter – alerts the audience to the complicated, subjective nature of cancer comedy. The glittering splendour of Carter's bath and his singing to an upbeat, exultant soundtrack clash with his wife's desperate anxiety. Two contradictory perspectives on cancer and comedy are brought together, making those watching aware of both the potential value and danger of this kind of comic relief.

In the focus groups I coordinated on this film, discussion of these two conflicting perspectives provided evidence of the highly subjective nature of humour about cancer. But it also illustrated how discussing cancer comedy films allows different opinions to be expressed and debated at a safe distance from real-world lives and relationships, and 'without judgement'.

This was shown in the debates that Carter's behaviour initiated. Whilst many participants responded positively to Cole and Carter's irreverent pursuit of laughter and joy, this behaviour was also the subject of disagreement in several focus groups. One participant argued that Cole and Carter's humorous, optimistic approach was 'true to life', because you must 'get rid of the negative people around you [if] their negativity is impacting you'. However, whilst this participant saw the film as portraying 'real life, the facts of it', another participant replied by insisting that Carter's decision to leave his wife behind and travel with Cole was 'a wee bit unreal'. Their disapproval was evident, as they compared Carter's actions to their own situation: 'you think that you're getting support from your other half, as we all do, but then he decides he's going to do his own thing'. This exchange demonstrated how a fictional narrative can draw out different opinions on incongruous, humorous approaches to cancer, as what appeared to show 'real life' for one individual was deemed 'unreal' and inconsiderate by another. And although each person involved in the debate alluded to personal experience, the films afforded a focus for the debate that enabled participants to disagree indirectly, through the fictional medium, rather than directly addressing one another's personal circumstances.

Cancer patients' experiences reveal the strange capacity for comedy to allow for a defiant acceptance of reality. As well as providing comic relief from the unpleasant truth of cancer, *The Bucket List* illustrates how humour can also offer patients a means of confronting truth directly in a humane, positive way. Many patients insist that despite its horror 'cancer cannot be sanctified' and 'some dark jokes are still very funny', even when they involve openly acknowledging the danger of this disease.[258] *The Bucket List* plays with this idea, testing the boundaries of taste and allowing viewers to begin to develop their personal, subjective understanding of which dark jokes can still be funny, and when. In Cole and Carter's screwball exchanges humour is frequently used as a vehicle for the truth. Their relationship could be used to support Rahner's claim about humour bringing us 'down to the truth',[259] as joking here serves as a means of facing cancer with honesty and humanity.

In *The Bucket List*, wise-cracking and truth-telling are often one and the same, as humour allows Cole and Carter to discuss their situation freely and strengthen their relationship. Analysis of the responses to this humour in the focus groups revealed how watching cancer comedy films can encourage those affected by cancer to reflect on the importance of a close connection when using humour. *The Bucket List* afforded examples that helped participants to convey the positive impact of humour within trusting relationships, as well as the value of environments in which they felt safe to share jokes. This was particularly noticeable in their responses to a scene in which Cole and Carter, sharing a hospital ward, discuss their treatments. As Cole waits anxiously for his first round of chemotherapy, he asks his friend what he should expect. Carter tells him that the treatment is 'not too bad, if you don't mind round the clock vomiting' or 'feeling like your veins are made of napalm', to which Cole responds sarcastically 'that's a relief'.[260]

Cole's deadpan responses point to a different kind of comic 'relief' at work here, which removes uncertainty and delivers truth with smiling, reassuring candour.[261] The tangible significance of the shared humour here is highlighted in real clinical trials, as patients who used joking and banter displayed an improved pain threshold and immune response, as well as 'elevations in natural killer cell activity' when reacting to tumours. Indeed, several participants suggested Carter's satire of chemotherapy implied a close connection between the two men, with one speculating that 'maybe the Morgan Freeman character had sussed out the Jack Nicholson character and feels he can say that' whilst another argued it showed that Carter understood Cole and thus was 'giving [the information] to him as he would speak'. Others stressed the importance of this 'sussing out' process, with one participant asserting that the way Carter joked about chemotherapy would only be appropriate 'if you knew the person very well, and they respond well to that kind of humour'.

The clip also helped many of the participants to explain how they feel humour can support and strengthen relationships, especially in reference to cancer support groups. Several participants linked Carter's use of humour to their own experiences of support groups, including one who said that 'it's like here [their support group], everyone has sussed out one another, and you know what you can say to one another'. A different participant compared Carter's use of humour to the shared 'cancer connection' at their group that meant they felt able to speak freely, 'like I can't talk to my family and friends'.[262] Watching the clip also encouraged participants to describe specific benefits of using humour within these groups. A participant who saw Carter's description of chemotherapy in a favourable light described Carter as someone 'further down the line in his treatment', who is guiding Cole in how to 'learn to live with it and cope with it'. Comparing it to their own experience, they said this 'reflects on everybody' because 'newly diagnosed people are all over the place', so need someone to help them 'settle down'. Interpreting the humour as a means of reassurance, the participant drew attention to the role they believed shared jokes can play in the mutual support and solidarity fellow patients provide. In a related observation, another participant suggested that Carter's use of humour had established a situation in which the two men could 'discuss things freely without being judged'.

Real patient stories sometimes describe a deathbed as a place where 'preciousness and pain' can be met with 'loving anecdotes and inside jokes', creating an atmosphere that is 'restful' and 'relaxed' as well as sorrowful.[263] A fictional exchange in *The Bucket List* reflects the comfort shared jokes can bring to those whose death is near. It suggests how acknowledging truth in the language of laughter could enable a patient to face dying with a confident smile, shedding tears mingling pain and joy.[264] In a scene close to the conclusion of *The Bucket List*, we witness this courageous, dignified humour shaping Carter's final moments. Having been hospitalised again and requiring dangerous surgery, we see Carter trapped in surroundings redolent of death. His frailty and hairless head are cruelly highlighted by harsh, uncompromising lighting, whilst his patient's gown and set details of drips, monitors and medical machinery deepen the foreboding, fatalistic feel of the shot. Into the murky morbidity steps Cole, with a smile on his face and a healthy dose of truth for his friend: 'you look like shit, Ray'. In the exchange that follows, Carter tells an amusing story about Cole's favourite brand of coffee which reduces the pair to tearful hysterics, allowing them to cross 'cry with laughter' off their bucket list.

Commenting on the scene at Carter's bedside, one participant in the focus groups argued that the upbeat tone established by Carter's use of humour was appropriate because 'if everything's got a sad ending, you feel miserable', whereas 'if you can laugh about it, it helps you to think positively about some of the things that have been talked about during the film'. If, as this implies, cancer comedy films could help people affected by cancer to entertain more positive perspectives on their situation, their potential value as humorous interventions is evident. Another participant described the scene as one that 'gives an uplift' because of Carter's joking: 'to think that he lay on that bed and how much he suffered, and yet he laughed and laughed'. Their response suggested that the clip afforded a boost to their mood and that, as well as encouraging positive patterns of thought, it could be used to improve a patient's emotional wellbeing. Carter's use of humour as he awaits life-threatening surgery also provides a fictional example of how humour can dissipate emotion in tense situations.

The playful entertainment *The Bucket List* presents also creates a space in which unorthodox, risky responses to cancer can be tested out.[265] By entertaining irreverent approaches to the problems cancer presents, *The Bucket List* makes possible this process of exploration, and therefore can allow people affected by cancer to consider the relevance of these approaches to their own situation.

Patients describe how a 'sense of fun' and willingness to exceed expectations for living with cancer helps them endure 'difficult treatments'.[266] Cole and Carter's pursuit of thrills and excitement invites the audience to become 'absorbed' in a playful probing of assumptions surrounding cancer.[267] The film contains characters, narratives and scenes that allow audiences to experience rediscovering 'freedom and flexibility' whilst coping with cancer, offering accessible entertainment that serves as a 'release from order and authority'.[268]

The Bucket List sets Cole up as a 'fool' determined to play his own game: a figure of fun who could introduce audiences to new ways of finding freedom and transforming their experience of cancer. This stubborn refusal to accede to the requirements of his surroundings takes on a new significance when Cole becomes a patient in a cancer ward. Even when his oncologist stands in front of Cole to give him the news that his diagnosis is terminal – 'a year if you're lucky' – Cole's immediate concern is that his view of the baseball game on the television is being obstructed: 'hey doc, you're blocking my view'. His insistence on focusing on entertainment and taking the game seriously adds absurdity and comedy to a tragic, shocking announcement.[269] Cole's refusal to take seriously his prognosis is indicative of the control he has reassumed over the course of his life with cancer, revealing the power his comic vision has granted him. This form of power was also revealed in the real-life story of a comedian Sarah-May Philo who 'made up songs' and 'cracked jokes' during awake brain surgery to 'break the ice'. She was able to use humour to change the 'atmosphere' of the operating theatre into a scenario 'like being in a café with your friends', transforming a traumatic procedure into an uplifting occasion and amusing story.

Viewers are alerted to the transformative power of this perspective by the symbolism of the bizarre glasses Cole is using to watch the baseball, which resemble two periscopes designed to allow him to remain lying horizontally. [270]

Whilst Cole's apparent indifference might appear absurd, one participant in the focus groups said they could 'identify very strongly' with Cole during the scene. Relating how they had often felt like 'somebody on the outside looking in at me getting all this treatment', the participant said they could 'identify with the way he's just more interested in the ballgame'. As these comments imply, patients with advanced cancer frequently list 'enjoying life' and 'engaging in meaningful activities' as key 'unfinished business themes',[271] so it is common for people in their position to feel deeply dissatisfied with 'a cure-driven biochemical model that regards their illness as a 'failure''.[272]

However, this scene also prompted those in the focus groups to reflect on the use of humour as a means of concealing feelings and deflecting attention. Several participants interpreted Cole's response to his prognosis in this light, with one suggesting that he behaved in a flippant, dismissive manner to his oncologist because 'he didn't want to show his emotion'. Developing this point, another participant compared Cole's reaction to their own response to diagnosis: 'when I first got told, my friend was with me and she had more of a reaction'. The participant said their instinct had been 'to deflect and put more focus on my friend, just like what he [Cole] was doing', comparing the clip to their own efforts to avoid attention. Other participants said they could 'relate' to this, speaking about their experiences of 'denial', or their initial refusal to 'acknowledge' or 'accept' their diagnosis.

The use of humour to conceal emotion was also the focus

of a discussion in another group, in which a participant commented on the impact of Cole's diagnosis scene. They thought that Cole was motivated by a 'fear of showing emotion, especially in front of other men'. Whilst saying they would have been in 'floods of tears' in Cole's position, the participant thought the scene 'was actually more powerful than if he had got upset'. The scene enabled the participant to understand better a form of emotional response that would not have come naturally to them.

Another fascinating aspect emerged when a participant raised the idea that using humour as a 'defence mechanism' was a 'male thing'. Referring to their experience as a healthcare professional, they said that 'having nursed ... I tended to find that men use this as a defence mechanism, because they find it so difficult to be open and honest'. By raising the notion that men 'will often use humour' in place of emotional candour, the participant revealed how comedy clips can afford starting points for difficult – and potentially divisive – discussions required to understand patients' and carers' attitudes to humour. Yet it was notable that, in other groups, women as well as men talked about being able to relate to Cole's use of humour to 'deflect'.

Cole and Carter's 'bucket list' plan becomes an exploration of the significance of comic foolery in the context of life with cancer. This is made explicit in an exchange between the pair when Carter admits he is worried that their scheme will lead him to 'make a fool of [himself]'. Cole's response – 'never too late' – is decisive in framing their journey as an investigation into the avenues that folly can open. The appeal, but also the danger, of their foolishness is captured in a crucial series of scenes which mark the beginning of their bucket list mission. When Carter explains their plans to his wife, Virginia, she responds with anger and confusion, calling her husband 'a fool who thinks he's figured out a way how not to have cancer', and asking him how he can 'just give up' and 'quit fighting' instead of trying experimental treatments. Motivated by her experiences as a nurse, Virginia is desperate to seek 'another opinion' on her husband's condition. It is easy to understand the pain of someone who feels alienated by this folly, and whose concern for her husband precludes joyful involvement in this radical scheme. Her distress is moving and relatable, yet the audience has already witnessed Cole, the Fool with Cancer, taking hold of her husband's imagination. As Virginia leaves, the lens captures Cole lurking in the back of the shot wearing a mischievous grin: a visual acknowledgement of this achievement. And, when the film cuts from Cole and Carter in the ward, dressed in hospital clothes, to the pair in a plane preparing to skydive, the editing creates a dramatic shift in tone and setting which further underlines Cole's success.

Evidence from the focus groups reveals how the film successfully captures and holds together two conflicting perspectives, affording an important opportunity to discuss the role that humour and folly should play in the life of a cancer patient. In several focus groups, Carter's dispute with his wife, Virginia, became the subject of a debate about whether his behaviour was 'selfish'. One participant said that they 'admired' Carter for 'taking that step to put [himself] first', arguing that his actions were justified because 'every day is a bonus for anybody that's been given a diagnosis'. But another participant took issue with this, saying that 'in Carter's situation' they would have 'explained about the bucket list' and invited their spouse 'to come along', because 'if they are in love ... they should build things together'. The film established an environment in which this emotive subject – that clearly felt relevant to several participants – could be discussed with relatively little risk of causing distress or offence. Participants could imagine how they would act in the same position, thinking about and talking through the issues in the hypothetical manner that the film made possible. One advantage of this emerged when the participant who 'admired' Carter's stubbornness, having heard the response their comments elicited, subsequently softened their position. Whilst maintaining that Carter 'committed his life at the right time and for the right reasons', they conceded that 'it's hard not to see it from both sides'.

The clip featuring Carter's wife also gave some participants an opportunity to bring a healthcare professional's perspective into the dialogue. Relating to the wife's position, one participant said that – as a nurse – they could understand Virginia's frustration, 'because nurses never like to think that they are somebody who's given up'. This observation brought to light one reason that a caregiver might find it difficult to reconcile themselves to an irreverent, incongruous attitude to cancer. By identifying with a fictional character, the participant was able to explain these concerns to other group members affected by cancer, in a safe environment set apart from the realities of a cancer ward. A different participant also chose to comment on this clip 'as a nurse', saying they felt that Carter's plans were 'a little bit unrealistic', as 'the nurse in me being protective would want him to do a bucket list that does not put extra pressure on [his health]'. Healthcare professionals usually find it easier to discuss matters relating to a patient's spiritual care indirectly,[273] and these responses revealed how cancer comedy films can be used to raise sensitive issues without directly addressing a patient's personal circumstances.

The Bucket List gives the imagery of levity and flight a central role, emphasising the uplifting qualities of comedy that can change our perspective on difficult experiences. Cole and Carter's flights around the world mean the audience – through the eyes of these fictional characters – can 'look down' on cancer, as cinematography captures the 'transcendent perspective' humour can bring: the means, as Gavin Hopps argues, of denying worldly affairs' 'ultimate seriousness'.[274] Once their flights are over, the protagonists are returned to matters of life, disease and death, but with a transformed perspective. Their journeys represent how humour can lift us out of difficult realities before placing us back down in the World of Cancer with a renewed vision of hope.

The Bucket List imagines how humour can make this kind of journey possible, drawing its protagonists out of the unforgiving setting of the cancer ward before returning them to it emotionally and spiritually changed. The very first item on their bucket list – skydiving – sees Cole and Carter flying high above the ground looking down at the distant earth below: an inescapably clear evocation of the 'transcendent perspective' their new game has given them. As they use Cole's private jet to travel between different exotic locations this imagery recurs, the emphasis shifting each time. Passing over an 'indescribably beautiful' polar ice-cap, the snow and ice glinting blue in the moonlight, this breath-taking shot moves the pair to begin a discussion about fate and faith. Their elevated position lets them appreciate the world with wonder and curiosity, provoking spiritual reflection as they fly suspended safely above the dismal daily grind of cancer treatment.

Yet the film portrays this journey as a temporary escape, rather than a permanent departure. A sudden change in tone, signalled by a switch to a calm, reflective soundtrack, marks their return flight to America and their lives as dying cancer patients. The audience is brought back down to earth by this shift in tone, as the influence of levity on the film's atmosphere and action recedes. However, in what follows, the film's conclusion makes evident the indelible mark their flight has left. Carter displays a newfound alertness to the joy his life contains, captured laughing amidst his family in a scene that visibly glows with warmth and merriment. As his wife puts it, Carter 'left a stranger and came back a husband': a character redefined by joy and humour. Cole, meanwhile, is now able to make a speech at Carter's funeral relating how 'deeply proud' he feels in the knowledge that he and Carter 'brought some joy to one another's lives'. The scriptwriters are at pains to emphasise the new meaning each has found during their travels and brought back into their everyday lives. Having flown above these normal existences and seen them from a 'transcendent perspective', they are no longer oppressed by the gravity of their condition.

The Bucket List does not simply leave the audience to interpret the role of levity in this process for themselves; rather, it offers Dante's *Divine Comedy* as an interpretative framework through which to understand Cole and Carter's journey. This is achieved through the enigmatic speech referenced at the start of this chapter, in which Cole is shown asking a collection of confused colleagues in a boardroom meeting if they have 'ever read the *Divine Comedy*'. An awkward silence, during which the camera picks out the baffled faces of Cole's staff, ensures the audience takes full notice of this strange question. Although there is no explanation given, the implication appears to be that Cole – as he tries to make sense of his time with Carter

– is starting to see their adventure as a recreation of Dante's mystical voyage from the 'spiritual gravity' of hell to the 'levity' of paradise, leading them towards the 'joy' residing at the 'heart of reality'.[275] Cole's mysterious question seems to redescribe his own journey as a secular reworking of this discovery of joyful transcendence. A crucial feature of the *Divine Comedy* is that, ultimately, it returns Dante to his original point of departure, but with a new vision of 'at least one telling spark' of divine glory to share.[276] Cole casts himself as the spiritual guide who has lured Carter out of the grounded, horizontal world of a car mechanic, introducing him to the heady heights of private air travel and a luxurious life full of mischievous joy. His words invite the audience to consider their bucket list exercise in light of the *Divine Comedy*'s pattern of flight and return, which places those involved back in their familiar reality with their spiritual perception transformed by a 'telling spark'. Cole and Carter's version of this process could make new audiences – who may never have 'read the *Divine Comedy*' – aware of the power of levity to transform the way we see ourselves and our lives.

This power of levity was evident in instances where the comical reframing of terminal cancer as an 'opportunity' in *The Bucket List* encouraged my focus group participants to explain their own outlook and decisions, and even appeared to prompt some to reconsider their life plans. Discussions around this theme were predominantly based on the crucial scene in which the list is created. After Cole and Carter are both given a poor prognosis and short life expectancy, they begin to discuss the things they would like to do before dying. Cole's comic vision leads him to reject the prospect of living his final months as 'a ceremonial procession into death', telling Carter instead: 'we got a real opportunity here'. Dismissing Carter's first draft of a bucket list as 'extremely weak', Cole gives it a 'little rewrite', devising a plan for them to go out 'guns blazing' and 'have some fun'. In reference to this, one participant said that Cole showed why you 'sometimes need somebody else who is pushy or blatant or bold' to 'get you to see something differently'. Another participant characterised Cole as a 'risk taker' who does 'outrageous' and 'extreme things', in contrast to Carter, who 'had his family and a different perspective on life'. Seeing Cole's influence on Carter led participants to reflect on the 'need' – in certain circumstances – for humour highlighting alternative, unconventional approaches to living with cancer.[277]

Although treating terminal cancer as an 'opportunity' will provoke anger in some patients, several participants in the focus groups found this captured their perspective. One reflected on the clip by saying 'that sounds great, a bucket list. Do the things you want to do, see if you can sneak in a few more holidays'. This profoundly positive appraisal was echoed by another participant, who approved of Cole's desire to seize an opportunity: 'I just want to fit in as much as I can while I can, I don't want to be two or three years down the line and say: "I wish I'd done that, and now I can't"'. The film's narrative appeared to capture many participants' motives and reflecting their desire to act with freedom in actively pursuing meaningful, pleasurable activities. The capacity for the clip showing the creation of the 'bucket list' to affirm these feelings was especially apparent in the comments of a participant who spoke about the scene in terms of grief. Saying that 'watching the film resonates with me', they explained this was because their father had been unable to fulfil his 'expectations' before dying of cancer: 'that question was put to a doctor, about my dad's bucket list, but sadly he couldn't make that choice'. Describing how this ordeal shaped their response to Cole's scheme, the participant said, 'that's why I think when I look at it, why not go for it'. The film established an environment in which the participant felt it was appropriate to speak candidly about how grief influenced their perspective on irreverent, defiant ways of living with cancer.

In every group, the central 'bucket list' idea became the basis for an important conversation about how a cancer diagnosis can cause a significant change in perspective. Indeed, one participant said that they 'like the movie' because it 'rings bells with me a lot, as it's just like after my first diagnosis when my outlook on life was completely changed'. Their reaction implied a direct connection between what the film portrayed and their emotions following diagnosis. There were several related comments in each group, such as one made by a participant in irreverent, comic language strikingly similar to Cole's tone and diction: 'this [cancer] gives you a kick up the backside to go back into looking at the better things in life and not sweating the small stuff... it makes you think life's too short'. The clip proved sufficient stimulus for a meaningful, honest discussion of the impact of a diagnosis on individuals' lives, including those who were facing the same decisions as Cole and Carter. This was true of one participant who said they could identify with Cole because they also 'equate [being] sombre with giving up', adding, 'either you fight it [cancer] and live the best life you can, or you go into your shell and accept it and your life is finished'.

The bucket list scheme not only reflected participants' outlook and resonated with their experiences, as for some it appeared to provoke reappraisal of their plans. This was the case for the participant who related 'a couple of things that have come to my mind watching this [film]'. One was 'that I want to watch the [full] film', and the second that 'I want to revamp my bucket list and really go for it!'. Another participant also discussed revising their own bucket list in response to the clips. Referring to a list they had already compiled, the participant said, 'there are some things I didn't think I would be able to do... but I am an optimist, so why not?'.

Conclusion

Combining cancer and comedy is a risky business. Laughing at a disease that causes pain, distress and death ought never to be done casually or carelessly. A mistimed, misdirected joke can cause serious offence when cancer is involved so it is crucial to pay attention to person, place and context.

Allowing patients to explore cancer comedy vicariously, rather than risking damaging real relationships, would undoubtedly add a valuable dimension to cancer care. The evidence from focus groups reveals the importance of this aspect of care, as the films afforded opportunities for sensitive, subjective matters to be discussed in a safe, indirect fashion.

These kinds of films are also suited to addressing another problem cancer often causes: boredom. Cycles of cancer treatment and recovery are full of dull hiatuses which cannot be filled with anything that requires energy or activity.[278] Amusing films that are accessible and relatively undemanding are ideal for filling these gaps, providing interest and fun for patients from the comfort and safety of a bed or sofa. To transform a despondent patient's imagination, it first must be captured; infectious humour, enjoyable characters, and exciting action could easily take hold of their thoughts and attention. Here, entertainment value is not the secondary concern some critics treat it as, but the crucial factor. Spiritual insights and liberating perspectives could seem more appealing when conveyed in the language of laughter.

The connections between cancer, levity, and 'flying' should also be considered. Within contemporary culture, several other fictional accounts of living with cancer use the imagery of flying as an important element of their stories.[279] It appears that many authors and artists have chosen the symbolism of flight as a metaphor for the spiritual value of fiction which lifts audiences out of familiar behaviours and environments, then returns them with a revitalised sense of purpose and possibility. And revealing reference to Dante's Divine Comedy in the Bucket List helps to explain why. Evidence from my focus groups clearly showed how people affected by cancer were moved to reassess their situation or revisit their own bucket list plans as they discussed the film. That highlights the significance of the journey into which viewers are drawn.

Chapter 6
CANCER, EMOTION AND SENTIMENTALITY

This chapter is about the definition and dangers of sentimentality, but also the value sentimentality can hold for people affected by cancer. There is much disagreement about what exactly sentimentality is, and some people are very critical of what they see as any kind of sentimental approach to cancer. But it is only in the details of moment, place, and person that the value, or danger, of certain emotions is revealed. The popular response to sentimental cancer fiction suggests that this genre can be valuable for those affected by cancer. In this chapter I use detailed analysis of two such artworks – Elizabeth Berg's novel *Talk Before Sleep*, and the eighth series of the long-running television drama *Cold Feet* – to explain how sentimental artworks can be used to enhance the spiritual care of cancer patients.[280] Drawing on my qualitative research, I have seen how the right artwork can seem 'relevant', cathartic or affirming precisely because of its sentimental qualities.[281]

Within each of the diverse forms of literature about cancer, there is often a suspicion of 'sentimentality'. At its most extreme, this mistrust leads to declarations that – for patients – 'sentimentality is more life-destroying than good honest hate'.[282] Underlying such violent aversion is a laudable desire to deal directly and truthfully with cancer. 'Honest information' is the foundation of good spiritual care, because 'minimising uncertainty' by ensuring patients are aware of the facts of their situation contributes to the creation of hope and purpose.[283] Consequently, psychologist Bruce Charlton describes sentimentality as an 'important problem' in healthcare: an 'attitude damaging to the proper practice of medicine' reliant on 'wishful thinking' instead of effective treatment.[284]

These arguments against sentimentality in a healthcare context are reflected in criticism of the sentimentality of contemporary cancer fiction. In her study of fiction about cancer, Mary Deshazer notes that 'much popular cancer fiction exudes sentimentality'. She focuses on the ways in which certain novels have 'contributed to the sentimentality of the breast cancer marketplace', which meets consumers' desire for emotional, romanticised stories about cancer.[285] Similarly, Susan Sontag observes that people impacted by cancer are frequently confronted by 'sentimentalist fantasies concocted about [their] situation'.[286] She raises important concerns about the ways in which these fantasies influence us, suggesting that the 'most truthful way of regarding illness' is one 'purified' of sentimental stories and metaphors. Disapproval of this 'pink sticky sentiment' echoes the concerns of those warning against the corrupting influence of sentimentality in patient care.[287] In each instance, there is a clear conviction that the sentimentalising of cancer prevents honest communication and intellectual clarity.

Such arguments highlight however a significant problem of all criticism of sentimentality. Warnings against sentimentality are complicated by the fact that 'just what sentimentality is and why it is objectionable remains something of a mystery',[288] and this is particularly problematic because the range of ways in which sentimentality is understood and applied is so broad.[289]

There are three most common criticisms of sentimentality. The first of these criticisms is based around the claim that sentimentality is the 'misrepresentation of things' to evoke, or indulge, emotions.[290] Sentimental art, moreover, may reduce hope to 'nostalgia' by fashioning a world in which death holds no sway.[291] This reflects a justifiable anxiety about denial: the danger of losing sight of 'the unsentimental fact of the matter' that 'death will happen to us all'.[292] Sentimentality is thus often associated with a willingness to 'substitute a "saccharine" portrait of the world for what we all know to be the horrible realities'.[293]

A second, closely-related critique of sentimentality focuses on the manipulation of emotions. This is often directed against sentimental fiction which allegedly 'substitutes cheap manipulation of feeling for careful calculation of form or judicious development of character'.[294] The death of Little Nell, one of 'Dickens' syrupy creations', is often seen as a paradigmatic example of this artificial, inauthentic process.[295] Using pathos to prompt emotional outpouring is regarded as the preserve of a work which is 'negatively characterised as a mere 'tear-jerker'': blunt instruments designed only to tug on our heartstrings.[296,297]

A third form of criticism takes aim at the 'indulgent' subject: the audience with an appetite for sentimentality. Here, sentimentality means 'unearned emotion' that is undeserved yet still sought out and enjoyed.[298] This line of criticism originated in the period when sentimentality first came to be used as a pejorative term, after Oscar Wilde described the 'sentimentalist' as someone who 'desires to have the luxury of an emotion without paying for it'.[299] It is easy today to find sentimentality branded as a sign of 'poor taste' because it is 'cheap' and 'superficial' emotion.[300] Others suggest that sentimentality is wrong because it encourages us to 'squander too much emotional energy'.[301]

There has also been much criticism *of sentimentality* from a theological point of view, notably by Jeremy Begbie who advocated something called 'countersentimentality'. He criticises sentimentality as a 'deep, pernicious strand in contemporary culture' that 'the arts have played a leading part in encouraging'. Although he acknowledges that sentimentality is a 'somewhat sprawling concept', he argues that it is best seen as 'a disease of the feelings' manifested primarily in people and secondarily in the arts.[302] Begbie does important work highlighting the need to take suffering and pain seriously, avoiding what William Stringfellow refers to as 'the sentimentalization of pain in the experience of a particular person'.[303] His warning that Western modernity is inclined to react to the 'pain and losses of the world' through 'evasion and trivialisation' – matched by 'the exaggeration of what is good or pleasing', such as 'the benefits of medical advances' – is important.[304] However, the problem is that these insightful warnings are used to justify a sweeping dismissal of all sentimentality.

The first criticism Begbie raises is that the sentimentalist 'avoids appropriate costly action', enjoying the emotional gratification which feelings like sympathy bring without taking action to correct injustice or prevent suffering. Wilde characterises the sentimentalist as one who will not 'pay' for emotional expenditure, and Begbie uses this to explain their failure to take 'costly action'.[305][306] He believes that when emotions are not emulating Christ's 'love-in-action', that is 'revealed most intensively on the cross', they are empty of beauty and meaning.[307]

Begbie's sentimentalists are, therefore, also 'emotionally self-indulgent', as they are concerned only with 'the satisfaction gained in exercising their emotion'.[308] Begbie uses the novelist Milan Kundera's well-known definition of kitsch to convey this criticism: a scornful satire of the 'second tear' of the sentimentalist, which says '[h]ow nice to be moved together with all mankind', expressing the sentimentalist's pleasure at the impression their emotion makes on others.[309] Kitsch and other sentimental art makes possible this gratifying indulgence, facilitating what Begbie describes as 'a rich emotional experience that will screen out the darker dimensions of reality'.[310] He concedes that 'comforting and immediately reassuring' art 'may have its place in some contexts', without elaborating on this seemingly crucial point. However, Begbie maintains that because 'beauty at its richest has been forged through the starkness and desolation of Good Friday', sentimental art can – at best – offer a cheap imitation of true beauty.[311]

The third identifying trait of the sentimentalist, in Begbie's view, is their willingness to see the world through 'rose tinted spectacles', so that only the 'pleasing or undisturbing aspects of a situation' are visible.[312] But Begbie believes that 'turning the aesthetic into an anaesthetic' will ultimately lure us away from Beauty Itself, as 'there can be nothing sentimental about God's beauty'.[313] As an example of art which offers aesthetic anaesthetic, Begbie says it is 'almost impossible not to mention greeting cards' that treat death as a 'friend in disguise'.[314] To explain the dangers of the 'tendency towards premature harmony' such artworks encourage, Begbie uses a passage in Dostoevsky's *The Brothers Karamazov* (1879) regarded as 'the classic wrestling with these matters in modern times'.[315] In his reading of this conversation between brothers Ivan and Alyosha Karamazov, Begbie argues Ivan's impassioned insistence that '[t]oo high a price has been placed on harmony' captures his own objections to theodicies reliant on the notion of an 'aesthetically harmonised final bliss'.[316] Ivan refuses to accept the idea that a beautiful resolution could compensate for all pain: '[s]urely I haven't suffered simply that I… may manure the soil of the future harmony for somebody else'.[317] And Begbie interprets Ivan as a voice for the fury felt by those, such as cancer patients, who face horrendous ordeals only to be told their pain is part of a higher plan 'contributing to the overall "beauty" of God's purposes'.[318]

In alluding to *The Brothers Karamazov* to support his view, Begbie ironically draws attention to a novel presenting a radically different theology of sentimentality. There is indeed another passage in Dostoevsky's novel that deals more directly with suffering and sentimentality. In the latter parts of the novel, Dostoevsky introduces the character of Kolya Krassotkin, an 'extremely vain' boy who detests displays of what he calls 'sheepish sentimentality'. Kolya intentionally avoids 'demonstrations of feeling' and is even suspicious of his mother's affection. His 'positive hatred' of sentimentality also leads him to treat his classmates with derision when they visit their dying friend, Ilusha. These visits are a 'great consolation to Ilusha in his suffering' but Kolya's aversion to all 'softness and sentimentality' means he feels unable to take part. Dostoevsky presents Koyla as an exaggerated parody of the kind of rationalising which treats open emotionality as indulgence. Behaving like someone who has swallowed whole an absolutist condemnation of sentimentality, Kolya reveals how easily such a stance can outgrow itself when accepted uncritically, casting doubt on all freely expressed feelings, however sincere.

What Dostoevsky's fictional exploration of sentimentality-in-practice exposes is the gap between academic debate and '"real life" emotional discrimination'.[319] It reveals that what happens at 'street level' is often overlooked by the 'highly literate minority who tell us that sentimentality is a dangerous corruption'.[320] A tendency to 'reject sentimentality as an expression of inferior, ill-bred being', sometimes used in male society to 'demean the emotionality of women',[321] appears to motivate Kolya's condescension. Kolya reflects some of the prejudices which can lurk behind objections passed off as purely intellectual criticism. This vain, prideful teenager, obsessed with appearing 'manly' and 'strong', is arguably emblematic of 'Western culture's difficulty with sentiment' – a difficulty which 'results in the shedding of tears, especially by men [being] seen as a negative, a psychological weakness'.[322] Kolya's conflation of 'emotionality with ineffectiveness'[323] speaks to the 'fear or condescension towards feeling' influencing contemporary Western culture.[324] This fear can push people towards extreme anti-sentimentalist positions, which do not allow for the subtleties and inconsistencies of our emotional lives.

The danger of these denunciations is that they ignore the potential value of sentimentality. Like other displays of heightened emotion, crying can be a natural and necessary means of expression. The kinds of 'self-conscious emotions' like empathy, guilt or grief which crying conveys are vital to the repair of social relationships,[325] whilst expressing positive emotions can ease human interactions and reduce stress.[326] Sentimentality can also be 'empowering', because it gives us a means of 'exploring and expressing desire',[327] bringing to mind those things we most urgently want or need. Sentimentality thus has a 'crucial place' in our lives because it 'keeps people in touch with their emotions',[328] confronting us with the griefs and joys which we might otherwise leave hidden. It can reconnect us with what lies beneath the polished surface of 'rational', tightly controlled behaviour, enabling us to overcome 'the collective repression of that which [our culture] finds uncomfortable'.[329]

Cancer patients' descriptions of the role sentimentality plays in their lives often provide a very different perspective to academic criticism of sentimentalism. Realism and directness are equally important aspects of spiritual care, but patients' testimonies suggest that 'indulging in easy emotion' is sometimes integral to the search for meaning. Indeed, cancer support specialist Dolores Morehead notes that a culture of 'being strong' denies those affected by cancer 'permission' to share their feelings, as it implies that 'to show emotion is a sign of weakness'.[330] To suppress all sentimentality is to 'stifle emotions that reassure people of their human value'.[331] I want to describe three areas of cancer patients' experiences – of 'healthy denial', of emotional release, and of 'simple' emotions – that reveal the potential value of sentimentality to those living with cancer.

Prolonged dealings with a hard, painful reality often leave cancer patients in need of the respite that sentimentality can bring. Physician and cancer survivor Dr Wendy Harper describes how she disliked being asked repeatedly about her cancer, because it 'undermined the distraction and healthy denial that minimised her distress'.[332] 'Healthy denial' also proved vital for a dying patient, who often acted in clear awareness of 'the true nature of her illness', but also 'resorted to a little make-believe on some occasions', using 'consoling day-dreams' to find relief.[333] As Hinton notes, '[t]here is no reason why [patients] should not have the comfort of make believe'; for someone who knew the truth, 'there was no need to diminish her remaining life by perversely brooding on death'.[334] The key distinction is between the forms of 'temporary but needed denial' described here (brief respite from emotional and physical pain), and the kind of violent, all-consuming, ceaseless denial practised by Walter White in Breaking Bad.

Psychoanalyst Halina Irving observes that it is natural for those with a 'grim cancer diagnosis' to 'go into some kind of denial', because if they thought about their illness all the time they 'could not go on living'.[335] This is why, as Nicholas Wolterstoff points out, we sometimes 'prize a work of art for its falsehood', when we 'want for a while to escape the drudgery and the pain, the boredom, perplexity and disorder of real life'.[336] While, from a healthcare perspective, Charlton contends that 'disease and death' are 'the least appropriate circumstances for indulging in evasion',[337] this overlooks those patients for whom 'indulging' in fantasies is a crucial coping mechanism.

Patients' stories also bring to light the importance of emotional release: the letting go of pent-up emotions that sentimentality can provoke. Objections to sentimentality are often connected to the assumption that 'crying is the fault of the crier', says Laura Otis, so that 'wails of anguish may be dismissed as bouts of weakness and self-indulgence'.[338] Cancer patients mention 'negative comments' about crying made in support groups by those processing sorrow and shock,[339] but suppressing such strong feelings increases stress levels, impairs memory and makes social interaction more difficult.[340] After being given a frightening prognosis, one patient found herself outside the hospital 'crying her eyes out'. When her family joined her, they all 'stood hugging each other and crying', as the most natural way of conveying love, support, and grief.[341] By letting her sadness and emotional fragility show, the patient revealed something that her family could share in and affirm. To an extent, this is akin to the shedding of the 'second tear' Kundera sees as epitome of sentimentality, in that it is the shared quality of these sentiments which means they serve as a source of gratification. It is only because the patient's emotions made an impression on her loved ones, moving them to join her, that this became an encouraging, meaningful experience. And, when people refuse to show signs of their emotional pain, it can be frustrating and dispiriting. One cancer patient speaks about the distress caused by her husband, who 'felt he had to be "the man" and not get emotional', when she needed him to 'cry with [her]' and 'let [her] have that feeling'.[342] Although it seems unlikely that Kundera's satire was intended to discourage the kind of affirmation this patient desired, criticism of sentimentality based on the impression externalised emotions make on others could easily be misinterpreted as an endorsement of being 'the man' and remaining coolly dispassionate.

There are many examples in patient testimonies of moments of simple tenderness that are extremely important. Medical journalist Lori Hope found that, having been asked to attend an urgent consultation with her oncologist, her mind 'was a washing machine spinning through cycles of worry'. She was 'vulnerable, desperately in need of nurturing, kindness, and comfort', and says that to have been offered a hug at that instant would have 'meant the world' to her.[343] There are times when natural, uncomplicated actions can bring peace and reassurance in a way that fulsome engagement with 'the complexities and ambiguity that evil brings' cannot.[344] '[A] big hug can mean everything when you're vulnerable',[345] said one Barts cancer patient, but there is not necessarily room for this kind of meaning in a strict 'countersentimentality'.[346]

Cumulatively, this range of testimonies indicates that abstract concepts of sentimentality will not always be the best means of understanding or evaluating our emotions. As soon as emotions are treated as embedded in real lives and interactions, we realise '[e]very emotion has its context, its implications, its place in our personality'.[347] Patients' stories show us that sentimentality, understood in terms of 'healthy denial', emotional release, and simple tenderness, is 'part of life'.[348][349]

The conversation should no longer be about what sentimentality is, or whether it is ethically or aesthetically suspect, but instead turns to the way features of the artwork resonate with each beholder. And this is the point at which the relationship between sentimental fiction and cancer starts to make sense. Artworks such as *Talk Before Sleep* or *Cold Feet* that bring to the surface supressed emotions, eliciting a response which releases pent-up feelings, or allows for tears to be shed, can be recognised for the value they hold for people living with cancer.

Reviewers of *Talk Before Sleep* bemoaned Berg's creation of a 'sappy tale' that was 'sentimental' and 'disappointing'.[350] Her depiction of the fictional relationship between Ann and her friend Ruth, who is dying of cancer, was denounced as typifying the 'ultrafeminine' and 'infantilising' themes of 'mainstream cancer fiction', contributing to the 'sentimentality' of commercialised cancer culture.[351] Indeed, it has been taken by some critics as a continuation of an unfortunate tradition that began with Little Nell: 'a late twentieth-century revision of the sentimental novel', in which 'domesticity, romantic attraction, and death from cancer converge'.[352]

If you come to sentimental fiction expecting stark realism and show no interest in the extent to which it invites emotional involvement you are missing the point.[353] By pursuing emotional realism, Berg created a work of fiction that could speak to the impact of cancer on our feelings and relationships. *Talk Before Sleep* is beloved by many readers, who have clearly found something meaningful in its pages. It received rave reviews from many popular sources[354] and is a *New York Times* bestseller averaging almost four stars (out of five) from over ten thousand ratings on goodreads.com.[355] It is clear from public reviews that many readers 'applied the book's lessons to their family experiences of cancer'.[356] Berg wrote *Talk Before Sleep* after losing a close friend to cancer, and describes her work as motivated by a desire 'to write about [her] experience in a fictional way', creating characters and events that 'although imagined, would testify to the emotional truth of what happened'.[357] And the sentimentality of *Talk Before Sleep* is integral to the opportunities to engage with the 'emotional truth' of cancer the novel affords. The *Book Reporter* review argued that Berg's experience of losing a friend to cancer 'afforded her a personal insight' that 'further enhanced her tender portrayal' of the intimate moments shared by the novel's protagonists.[358] One reader describes how *Talk Before Sleep* 'stirred all [her] emotions' after her mother in law was diagnosed with cancer, saying the novel 'made it a little easier to face the reality of it all'.[359] [360]

The potential relevance of Berg's novel for someone in this position was also highlighted by a participant in my Fiction Library trial. Referring to their personal experiences, the participant described how they found *Talk Before Sleep* to be a 'helpful' source of affirmation:

> I sadly lost my best friend to bowel cancer three years ago ... I really related to Ann, how hard it is to lose

someone so close. I too went through stages of anger. This book would be particularly helpful to someone looking after a loved one at the end of their life.

Invited to comment on the sentimental qualities of *Talk Before Sleep*, one participant in the focus groups also spoke about the role their personal experiences played in shaping their interpretation of the novel. Observing that 'everybody's journey is personal', they added that 'having had cancer in the family from a young age [and] working in palliative care, combined with my character and personality and how I see things, maybe I read this book in a way related to that'. Responding to these comments, another participant described a powerful, poignant example of this kind of interaction with an artwork:

> I had very mixed feelings when I was reading it. I related to it, as I also suffered from breast cancer. So although I'm in the clear, you know, secondary cancer is always at the back of my mind... So, in the beginning of the book, I struggled a bit, I actually nearly just put it down, then wanted to finish it... I know it is a true story, but it is just too close to home. I wasn't comfortable within it... So, yeah, I had really deep emotions about this book.

It clearly felt natural to these participants to discuss the novel in terms of their individual circumstances and emotions, in order to convey the complex interplay between their personal perspective and the affective, sentimental qualities of the work.

The same approach will help to highlight the meaning viewers found in the eighth series of *Cold Feet*, which portrays Jenny Gifford's fictional experiences of cancer with warmth and sentimentality. Some reviewers criticised this central storyline. Jasper Rees describes it as 'mortality lite': an insubstantial narrative about cancer that played out with 'pendulum-like reliability'.[361] Sean O'Grady saw the series-eight revival as a 'silly' fiction that 'belongs in the past', and was full of 'irritating and painful moments'.[362] Developing this theme of a dated, anachronistic series, Thomas Sutcliffe compares *Cold Feet* directly to the Death of Little Nell in Charles Dickens' The Old Curiosity Shop and its 'Victorian sentimental excess'. However, he also acknowledges that, whilst the series' emotional plotlines would be easy to dismiss as 'morbid indulgence in sentiment', the popular reception of *Cold Feet* revealed how television could create characters who occupy an 'important psychological space in people's lives', blurring the distinction between the 'stories we inhabit' and the 'stories we watch'.[363] Despite some unfavourable critical assessments, this was a show that 'struck a chord' with many people and 'moved viewers to tears'.[364] The actress Fay Ripley, who plays Jenny, describes how she is frequently approached by strangers with real experiences of cancer because of the ways her character's fictional story reflected theirs: 'they want to come up, introduce themselves and tell me their story'.[365] This was underlined by a participant in my Fiction Library trial with cancer patients, who explained that the 'thoughts and feelings' that Ripley (as Jenny) conveyed felt familiar to them: 'I, like Jenny, have experienced breast cancer [and] it was portrayed very well. The thoughts and feelings that I had were very similar to those of Jenny, especially the fear'. Their comments are illustrative of the connection between Jenny's storyline and the real-life affective impact of cancer that was apparent in the public response.[366]

Several reviewers noted the vital role the series'

sentimentality played in establishing this connection. Sarah Hughes described the final episode as a 'sentimental and perfectly pitched finale': the conclusion to a piece of 'warm, comforting television' that 'accurately reflected the reality of life for many people'.[367] The idea that an artwork could be warm, comforting and sentimental, whilst also reflecting accurately aspects of the powerful and painful reality of cancer, seems to contradict arguments against sentimentality made on the basis of its deceptive, manipulative nature. And yet, this does appear to reflect how many viewers saw the series. Notably, professional cancer support specialists picked up on the series, promoting Jenny Gifford's fictional journey as one which captured the 'strange emotional landscapes' of cancer and could draw out 'emotions that many people don't always acknowledge'[368]

In what follows, I explore how works like *Talk Before Sleep* and *Cold Feet* can illustrate how becoming 'caught up' in sentimental fiction could allow those affected by cancer to: i) recognise emotional suppression; ii) appreciate the 'importance of crying'; iii) embrace emotional openness; iv) find respite from difficult realities; and v) discern new, consoling meaning within their experiences.

Fictional, sentimental stories of cancer offer narratives in which audiences can find their own tendencies towards emotional suppression reflected, identifying with signs of secrecy and shame which resonate with their personal experiences. *Talk Before Sleep* shows critical awareness of the all-too-familiar culture of concealed emotions in which any sign of 'aroused sentiment' is, observes Clive Marsh, 'seen as a negative, a psychological weakness'.

When Ann and Ruth first meet, a fleeting moment of emotional identification draws them together — a moment in which the burden of buried emotions is briefly shared.

Chatting over a meal, Ruth starts to discuss her struggling marriage, and Ann notices she is 'close to tears', watching 'her hands flutter, mothlike, around her face, ready to wipe away the evidence of her grief'. Although she does not acknowledge it, Ann relates to her new friend's feelings, recalling the 'tears of a terrible and too-familiar loneliness' she had shed the night before. Despite this recognition, all Ann can offer in response is a fatuous truism concealing her true reaction: 'I know marriage has its ups and downs', whilst Ruth, in turn, 'acts perfectly fine and friendly' the moment she is back in her husband's company. The narrative switches between candour and concealment, private truth and outward deception, using the movements into and out of Ann's interior monologue to dramatise the disconnect between what each woman feels, and what they are willing to reveal. They understand one another's loneliness but share an impulse to hide 'evidence' of their sentiments. This impulse gave a form of affirmation to a participant in the focus groups who recognised the two women's instinctive fear of showing emotion: 'I kind of pick up on that bit about being embarrassed for people to see me because I am an emotional person. But I'm always apologising to people for crying'. This sentiment was echoed by several other participants, such as one who described how this pressure to appear 'strong' can lead to forms of emotional self-neglect, saying that when 'you're trying to be brave for everyone else, then you forget about you as a person and what you're going through'). Evidently, the novel exposes a real culture of concealment that stigmatises open displays of grief, and can influence how cancer patients feel and behave.

Reflecting this fear of candour, Berg not only gives the reader a point of comparison for their own emotional landscape, but also links this fear to a specific aspect of life with cancer: its medical treatment. When Ruth visits her oncologist, Ann notices that he keeps an 'antiseptic distance' from Ruth, physically and emotionally, withholding information and avoiding meaningful contact. And in an even more unpleasant instance of this distancing, the radiology resident analysing Ruth's scans steps away after greeting her 'as though she were contagious'. She is regarded with 'something resembling fear mixed with pity' and finds her doctors 'hiding' from her, 'using the vocabulary of medicine' to avoid being honest and compassionate when they deliver bad news. The 'antiseptic' atmosphere of unsentimental rationality characterising Ruth's treatment seems to have influenced her response to the emotional turmoil cancer provokes.

Michael Bell argues that reading fiction can be 'an implicit form of emotional self-examination',[369] as we interpret characters in relation to ourselves, and to how we would feel in these imagined situations. This was the case for a participant in the focus groups who said that the passage describing Ruth's meeting with her oncologist 'resonated with me quite a bit'. Because they knew that they were likely to develop metastatic cancer in the future, the participant found themselves inhabiting Ruth's perspective: 'when I read that part, I was imagining myself being in that situation at some time in the future, so I had a sharp intake of breath reading that bit'. The participant described how they were 'relating' to Ruth's desire to appear 'strong', yet also with the sense of fear Ruth is concealing: 'deep down she knows she's in the final stages of her journey'. Responding to these comments, another participant also said they could 'relate a wee bit' to Ruth's situation. Describing how they had recently been in hospital for a scan, the participant explained they had felt 'a bit of fear' concerning the results, adding: 'sometimes I wish I could have had a bit more blunt conversation with my surgeon'.

In both cases, participants were moved to reflect on the feelings that they had chosen to hide during their meetings with clinicians. These examples suggest that, if a reader of *Talk Before Sleep* found themselves identifying with Ann and Ruth's inclination to emotional reticence, noticing how it originated in the treatment room before spreading into their behaviour and relationships, their reading can become 'an exercise of "real life" emotional discrimination'.[370]

In *Cold Feet*, the ensemble cast enables the series to explore emotional suppression from varied perspectives, creating scenarios which could resonate with different forms of concealment in viewers' lives. The form most relevant to those affected by cancer is Jenny's reluctance to tell her family about her diagnosis, and the way it is making her feel. Struggling to find the 'right moment' to announce her news, she keeps her anxieties hidden, searching for information on breast cancer in bed at night to maintain her deception, the glow of her smartphone illuminating a tense, troubled face.[371] In a particularly poignant scene, Jenny, still reluctant to tell her family the news of her diagnosis, is left alone in the shadows at the foot of the stairs in her family home, listening to receding voices discussing plans for her daughter's eighteenth birthday party, which she fears she may not live to witness. The fading conversation represents the distance Jenny's secrecy is beginning to create between her and her loved ones, as they become separated from her private 'emotional truth'.[372]

This theme of concealed emotion is picked up in other storylines across the series, showing its relevance to a range of relatable, everyday situations. Adam (James Nesbitt) is accused of being a middle-aged father who is 'not ready to grow old', 'scared to death' of his own mortality. His 'sad and totally pathetic behaviour' – chasing younger women – is a sign of an unwillingness to admit his concerns as he conceals his emotional fragility under a mid-life crisis. Meanwhile David (Robert Bathurst) is prevented by pride from asking his friends for help as he is plunged into financial difficulties. Eventually, after putting on a 'brave face' and hiding his troubles, he is left alone in a carpark in pouring rain, the camera panning out from above on his solitary, soaked figure, whilst a mournful voice sings 'where do we go from here?'.

The series is all about how 'we' move beyond secrecy and shame: how Adam, David, Jenny – but also the viewer – can overcome barriers to honest emotional expression. A montage at the start of the fourth episode ties together these storylines using brooding music with lyrics about internalised anxieties: 'I got guns in my head and they won't go', linking Jenny's concealment to problematic cultural ideals of stoicism and bravery. [373]

Sentimental artworks are not just there for audiences unsure of their feelings, seeking to uncover buried emotions, as they also afford opportunities for emotional release to those who know they need a means of unburdening. Whilst you are undergoing treatment for cancer, or recovering from its impact, it can be hard to find appropriate moments to release pent-up feelings. The calm, clean professionalism of a cancer ward, as well as the presence of strangers, is not conducive to free emotional expression. Yet, as Jenny's concerns about finding the 'right time' to tell her family illustrate, it can be just as difficult to find apposite moments to show strong feelings during domestic life. There is often an element of intentionality inherent in reading a sob-story or watching a tear-jerker – an active choice made by someone searching for an excuse to let go of their emotions – and this contract between beholder and artwork is crucial to understanding the meaning these works hold for those who seek them out.[374] Cancer patients may come, deliberately, to sentimental artworks to release all the emotions they feel they cannot show in an oncologist's office.

Dolores Morehead helps to explain exactly why the environment sentimental art creates can be valuable. She observes that 'patients need to be able to break down' and should be given 'permission' to do this,[375] and it is this 'permission' that sentimental art affords. Patient support groups and counselling sessions also provide a space for patients to release their feelings, but works like *Talk Before Sleep* and *Cold Feet* offer an alternative outlet for those who cannot, or choose not to, access these resources. The 'emotionally devastating' scene in *Cold Feet* in which Jenny finally confides in another person, her friend Karen, about her cancer is a perfect example of this. In this 'downright tear-inducing' moment, the viewer can 'feel [Jenny's] hurt and helplessness', as the concern Karen shows gives Jenny permission to let out all the powerful feelings that have accumulated.[376] As the camera slowly draws away from the two friends embracing, all sound is replaced by reflective music, offering the viewer stillness and time in which to share in this cathartic moment. It is interesting to note that Fay Ripley 'admitted she was sobbing real tears over her father' during this scene, as she found her own grief after a recent bereavement became 'easily accessible' while she performed it.[377] Her personal experience demonstrates that this fictional scene can invite the release of real emotion, making viewers' feelings 'easily accessible' by fostering an environment in which they feel they have permission to break down.[378]

CANCER, EMOTION AND SENTIMENTALITY

A shared love of sentimental films is one of the things that solidifies Ann and Ruth's friendship in *Talk Before Sleep*, as each understands the other's need for the catharsis these films afford. Ruth takes Ann to see *Sophie's Choice* (1982) and, as Ann's narration reveals, this classic of the tear-jerker genre provides exactly what they hoped for. Ann relates how she 'couldn't wait to cry', and how she thought the film was 'terrific' because it 'ripped your heart out and flung it on the floor'. When the film concludes, the pair are left 'overwhelmed with sorrow', with swollen eyes and faces 'splotchy with grief'. To underline that this is an experience they actively sought out, Berg includes the detail of Ruth coming armed with her grandmother's special handkerchiefs to wipe up the inevitable tears. The film created an environment in the cinema in which 'everybody was crying' and letting sorrow show was acceptable and even expected. Berg's fiction here makes the same point as Marsh, when he argues that crying at the cinema is an 'instructive, developmental and quite normal human experience'. Because 'sentimental, melodramatic films' provoke this experience, they are a key coping mechanism in a culture dealing with the 'collective repression' of certain types of emotion.[379] This passage prompted a participant in one of my focus groups to describe how they had learned that it is 'good to cry', and that 'every time [they] see someone cry' they encourage this, saying: 'don't feel embarrassed because it's a way of letting go, of expressing, because otherwise when you bottle up it's not going to do your mental health any good'. Through affording an illustration of the importance of 'letting go', the passage drew the participant into a discussion of what they had learned about the necessity of emotional expression. [380]

As well as providing moments which bring us into

touch with our emotions, *Cold Feet* and *Talk Before Sleep* give their audience opportunities for escape, prescribing sentimentality as a heartening distraction from grim realities. *Cold Feet* contrives contexts in which the value of 'aesthetic anaesthetic' comes to light, showing through Jenny's storyline how the 'protective function' of sentimental art can afford a 'therapeutic escape from pressure'.[381] [382]

While Jenny endures rounds of cancer treatment and gradually comes to terms with her situation, she is also seeking out fun. Her search for escapism leads her to agree to read the draft of a sentimental romantic novel, *Love Comes Slowly*, for her friend Karen (an editor). Karen is unimpressed, dismissing the novel as 'the sort of useless dross young women lap up when they could be thinking'. But Jenny realises the book is exactly what she is looking for, volunteering to read through the draft because she 'could do with a distraction'. Where Karen sees 'useless dross', Jenny recognises a source of sentimental escapism that could bring her respite from private anxieties. Karen cannot understand why Jenny would choose to 'lap up' this novel instead of something more intellectually challenging, because she is unaware of the circumstances pushing Jenny to find fiction which will allow her to 'pretend it's ok' for a few hours.[383]

As well as seeing Jenny enjoying this pretence, *Cold Feet* also invites viewers to join in with her fun in scenes as 'completely daft' as they are necessary. In one comic interlude, we discover that the author of *Love Comes Slowly*, 'Nina B. St James', is in fact an unassuming middle-aged man (played by Paul Ritter). The result of this plot-twist, which mischievously subverts expectations surrounding the assumed femininity of this genre – '*you* write romantic fiction?' – is that Jenny offers to become the public face of the author. Using extravagant wigs and garish costumes to create her alter-ego, she discovers playing the role of Nina is a perfect way to 'have a bit of fun', as – whilst Jenny is contending with chemotherapy and cancer – 'Nina's feeling just fine'. Silly, slapstick scenes combine a gurning Paul Ritter with the ostentatiously dressed 'Nina' striking ridiculous poses, giving the audience some joyously farcical light relief. A voice often heard in cancer patients' testimonies is that of the sufferer 'desperate to get out of hospital': the weary individual who 'wanted to be somewhere else' and 'escape' their situation for a while.[384] It is this voice Jenny is echoing when she implores Karen to let her maintain their elaborate deception: 'please don't leave me listening to the chemo running through my veins'. And, when she becomes Nina, engrossed in her act, Jenny gives herself and the audience a 'holiday from the real woes of the world'.[385]

Talk Before Sleep also offers readers a 'holiday' from the darker dimensions of reality. There is often an element of luxurious indulgence to the moments of relief Berg describes: scenes full of coffee and sweet treats in which Ruth, Ann, and their friends 'eat and laugh and talk, and nobody says anything about illness or death or dying'. Berg uses Ann's commentary to explain the value of these gatherings, that Ann cherishes because they are 'so close to the old way': a nostalgic revisiting of past pleasures affording time away from distressing subjects . The friendship group treat food as a source of escapism, and the reader's privileged access to Ann's thoughts reveal why this is precious to them.[386]

Ruth's romantic escapades also grant her, and the reader, relief from a painful present, as a pretext for scenes of sentimental escapism comparable to those created by Jenny Gifford's antics as 'Nina'. When an old flame appears, Ruth sees this as an opportunity to recapture the exhilaration of her youth. Again, it is Ann's observations which explain the welcome contrast this represents, dragging their attention – and the reader's – away from darker things: '[w]e've been talking codicils. We've been visiting graveyards. Now we've got to find Ruth's mascara so she can get ready for a date'. While Ann struggles to make sense of this sudden shift in tone, a brief exchange with another of Ruth's friends sheds light on the true value of this adventure. 'Is this real?', Ann asks, to which the response is 'what the hell difference does that make?'. In this context, what is 'real' or realistic is irrelevant, as it is the restorative respite from codicils and graveyards Ruth's date affords which gives her hopeless romantic fling its meaning. This pursuit of romantic escapism resonated with a participant in the focus groups who described themselves as 'a bit of a Ruth character', adding: 'since my first diagnosis ... my whole outlook on life is completely different'. They explained that this 'new outlook' meant that they simply followed their desire for excitement or adventure: 'I'm just like, I want to learn something, and I want to do something, and I will do it now, because I don't know what tomorrow holds'. Their self-designated 'couldn't care less' attitude was clearly reflected and affirmed in Ruth's pursuit of romance in defiance of the tragic reality of her prognosis.

In *Cold Feet* and *Talk Before Sleep* we see how sentimental art can play an important role in the Search for Meaning. The kind of generous, vague spirituality which sentimentality lends itself to is often what those in pain embrace. Where fraught questions of dogma and doctrine might feel too abstract, simple spiritual comforts offer an alternative. Focusing on the sentimental 'world of love, generosity, kindness, awe and wonder' involves setting aside the more challenging dimensions of life, but this can supply encouragement where it is urgently required, maintaining a connection to spiritual values of 'consciousness, cooperation and love'.[387] Sober rational reflection, whether scientific or theological, is not always the best way into personal experiences of suffering. *Cold Feet* and *Talk Before Sleep* give audiences a different mode of engagement: a sentimental spirituality in which hope and reassurance are not hard-won luxuries, but freely-given gifts.

In *Talk Before Sleep*, sentimentality is integral to the search for spiritual solace, as Ann and Ruth both seek out images of transcendence which will bring them peace. Mary Deshazer notes that the novel's 'discourse of salvation, faith, miracles and angels lends a religious tone to an otherwise secular novel'.[388] When Ruth is conveying her wishes for her burial, she asks for an angel to watch over her: 'I've been dreaming about angels. I think they're real. I want one on my grave'. As she nears death, Ruth's sense of what is 'real' is governed by this vision of an angelic guardian, because this is what brings her comfort. Theologians who advise against offering 'theological cotton-candy' to cancer patients would be unlikely to condone the 'melt-in-your-mouth' sweetness of this imagery,[389] but Berg shows why it will have a place in real people's experiences of cancer – such as the breast cancer survivor who explains that she 'wasn't a spiritual person' before her diagnosis, but now 'truly believe[s] in guardian angels'.[390]

Evidence from my focus groups also indicated that the seemingly sentimental talk of guardian angels can invite constructive engagement from people affected by cancer. The passage initiated conversations about participants' desire to plan for their death. This included one person who noted the similarity between Ruth's wishes and their own:

'I had a cousin who died suddenly at the age of 50. And I was at the funeral, I came home from that funeral, and I spent an hour writing down how I want the same situation as what Ruth has'. Others chose to speak about their own specific wishes, such as being buried rather than cremated, or having a scroll on their headstone. The emotional clarity and candour Ruth shows was a starting point for difficult discussions, opening a space in which participants felt comfortable talking honestly and directly about funerals and gravestones. One participant related how the passage had 'triggered' them to reflect on their wishes for death, and on the importance of conveying these: 'in the passage, I really liked that [Ruth] said "I want some control"... it just triggers me to think of what you want. And that you know, perhaps you need to remind others. Those are the hard conversations to have'. It appears that the soft, saccharine qualities of the novel's spirituality can ease patients into 'hard conversations' about death.

The sentimentality of Ruth's narrative also reveals how meaning can emerge amidst the darker dimensions of cancer, giving readers reassuring glimpses of 'awe and wonder'. This is especially apparent in an exchange between Ann and Ruth, in which Ruth tries to convey this strange intermingling of contrasting emotions. When Ann relates how she is 'glad' that Ruth can be 'peaceful' at certain times, Ruth responds:

> Oh yeah, when I'm not terrified, I'm real peaceful. And you know what else? It's such a rich thing. It's so... good. And sometimes I think, God, my life has taken these awful turns, but they're also sort of wonderful. I mean, the constant presence of you all – my friends.

This seems to be a scene full of sentimentality, in which spiritual values of 'cooperation and love' are emphasised whilst the 'awful' aspects of cancer fade into the background. So, it was unsurprising to find some participants in the focus groups reacting strongly to this portrayal of life with cancer as 'also sort of wonderful'. One participant objected to this description, saying it was 'definitely not [true] for me', adding: 'I would give anything not to have gone through the last six months', referring to their experiences of cancer. Yet other participants found Ruth's words captured familiar emotions, such as the participant who responded to Ruth's description of feeling 'terrified and peaceful' by saying: 'I think we've all experienced that'. This positive appraisal of Ruth's speech was shared by a participant who clearly felt that Berg's writing, which they were reflecting on alongside Hazel Grace's evocation of a 'little infinity' in *The Fault in Our Stars*,[391] had accurately described the 'emotional truth' of cancer. Relating how, as a healthcare professional, being diagnosed with cancer had changed their perspective, the participant said:

> I like that Ruth says 'when I'm not terrified. I'm real peaceful'. And that actually, for me, explains or really describes well how it can be like a rollercoaster ... And I think both passages for me, really explain how it's the dichotomy, if you like, of cancer, how it can be such a terrible thing and, you know, some people have said: 'Why me?' and all the rest of it, but actually, it can truly enrich your life. And that's not anything I expected at the time of my diagnosis. And I did have patients before that used to say to me: 'it's the best thing that's ever happened to me' and I'd look at them and think well, that's just plain weird. I wouldn't ever say it, but that I

could not understand that until it happened to me [a cancer diagnosis], and I know now exactly what they're talking about. So, I think these passages introduce that hidden aspect of it really well.

As this response reveals, the language Berg employed can offer resources and affirmation to someone seeking to 'explain' the 'rollercoaster' of cancer, as well as helping patients to access the 'hidden aspects' of living with cancer that might remain concealed and unacknowledged in a clinical context. Whilst, for a healthcare professional, the notion that cancer can be wonderful might appear 'weird', Berg's novel can enable a patient to recognise and speak about those moments when cancer can 'enrich your life'.

For a reader who has chosen *Talk Before Sleep*, sentimental spiritual encouragement is likely to be what they are looking for. Like those who bring anxiety and agony to popular devotional images, writes David Morgan, 'the transcendence they seek is deliverment from ailment and anguish'.[392] While Ann tries to reconcile herself to the prospect of losing her friend, she is searching for this 'deliverment'. When this search leads her to a psychic, the conversation does not follow along the lines Ann was anticipating. Trying to find words which fit her spirituality, Ann tells the psychic 'I don't exactly believe in God... I think what I believe in is a Great Spirit'. Yet when the psychic responds by challenging this distinction – 'Don't you know... That God *is* a spirit?' – Ann's search for meaning changes course. Later, passing a small Catholic church, she suddenly decides to enter and pray, telling the reader 'you try, sometimes, in spite of yourself'. Berg's narrative captures a vague, vulnerable spirituality seeking clarity and consolation: a tentative creed shaken by cancer and prefaced by 'I think', not 'I believe'.

The power of sentimentality to provoke spiritual healing is revealed in *Cold Feet*, most notably in its use of sentimental music to offer viewers space for reflection and recovery. In a significant exchange between Karen and a hospital chaplain, the spiritual distress cancer can cause is painfully apparent. The weary, embattled chaplain has just been rudely rebuffed by Jenny when he tried to comfort her before surgery. Shortly after, Karen comes across him assaulting the hospital coffee machine, having a 'temporary crisis of faith' as the machine steals his change, the culmination of what has clearly been a trying day. His theological training seems to have proven inadequate in the face of the suffering he encounters, and the ambivalence his offers of prayer are met with. Telling Karen stories of the heart-rending human tragedies he must respond to, the chaplain admits that sometimes 'the sheer weight of it' becomes too much to bear.

Like Ivan Karamazov, this is a man who wants to 'return his ticket' and receive a refund – from both the coffee machine and the Eternal Creator, as the visual metaphor implies. And yet, like Dostoevsky, the writers of *Cold Feet* do not leave things there, presenting a 'practical answer' to this theoretical problem of suffering. Later in the episode, we watch the chaplain, accompanied by Sharon van Etten's stirring song about troubled souls *Every Time the Sun Comes Up* (2014), finding the homeless, pitiful figure of David asleep on a hospital bench. Taking time to find a blanket to place over David, the chaplain displays what Rowan Williams has called that 'love in small particulars' rooted in everyday humanity which typifies Alyosha Karamazov's response to Ivan's challenge. Alyosha's practical, grounded commitment to such love provides the counterpoint to

Kolya's cold, absurd anti-sentimentalism, offering an alternative approach to the problem of sentimentality.[393] Easing the burden of suffering by responding to each individual with compassionate care, the chaplain turns to addressing emotional pain instead of trying to solve an abstract intellectual conundrum. Its meaning distilled by a moving melody and lyrics, this brief scene becomes part of the series' spiritual response to 'the sheer weight of it', balancing existential despair against sympathetic, sentimental images of spiritual care.

The way in which the interaction between an individual viewer of *Cold Feet* and the series itself creates new meaning is perfectly illustrated through the use of another sentimental song in the series finale. After her friend and fellow patient Charlie dies, Jenny participates in a concert with the choir for cancer patients Charlie persuaded her to join. In a tearful speech, Jenny dedicates the choir's final number to Charlie, describing how losing a loved one 'changes your perspective on things'. As she sings an arrangement of *Happy Together* – about enduring love – by The Turtles, her grief gives the melody and lyrics a new resonance.[394] But it is not only Jenny's experiences which are contributing to the meaning the music holds. While she sings, the camera moves between her friends and family in the audience, capturing different moments of affection and reconciliation: Adam's newfound closeness with his son; David reunited with his friends; Jenny's family supporting one another. Each time the shot switches, the lyrics of *Happy Together* take on a new significance and the upbeat, joyful tone and tempo of the music captures a different feeling. As viewers, we are asked to participate in the kind of communal, ritualistic meaning-making that can occur through the 'aesthetic effect of listening to a particular piece of music in a particular setting, with particular people'.[395] Every audience member seems to be finding their own emotions affirmed and enriched by what they are hearing, as the music 'receives meaning through interactions that are interpreted differently by each participant'.[396] In the environment created by the scene of Jenny's speech and song, deemed 'absolutely', unmistakably 'sentimental' by critics,[397] each listener is invited to find their own joy and consolation within the music.

Conclusion

This chapter proposes a new approach to sentimentality and cancer care. Romantic, sentimental stories about cancer have proven increasingly popular in recent times,[398] and academics should perhaps begin by asking not whether these are morally suspect, indulgent fantasies, but rather why so many people turn to them. Resisting the temptation to pronounce judgement on tear-jerkers without first trying to understand their appeal will bring academic research closer to the realities of lived experience.[399] Like spirituality, sentimentality is best used as a productively imprecise idea that can open an area of experience for exploration: a pliable concept ready to be reshaped in accordance with each individual's perspective. As the evidence from my qualitative research shows, sentimental fiction can give patients, friends, and families a new means of accessing and expressing their emotions, complementing the strictly reasoned realism of clinical care. This is what the warmth, generosity, and excess of sentimental stories like *Talk Before Sleep* and *Cold Feet* can provide. *Cold Feet* is also an illustration of the capacity for accessible, fictional narratives to be used to engage with an area of experience that contemporary healthcare, and society as a whole, struggles to address.

Interpreting these works in terms of how they might meet the emotional needs of those affected by cancer reveals why they 'struck a chord' with audiences, reflecting the 'emotional truth' of cancer. They offered 'aesthetic anaesthetic': targeted treatment for those seeking something more than grim realism and the 'stoicism' of stifled sobs.

FINAL THOUGHTS

In the latter stages of the nineteenth century, George Eliot used literary fiction to draw attention to the problem of spiritual care – a problem that remains unresolved today. In typically prescient fashion, Eliot satirised the increasingly apathetic, blasé attitude towards spiritual concerns identifiable within the medical professions in her novel *Middlemarch*. Through the character of the ambitious young doctor Tertius Lydgate, Eliot revealed how spiritual matters had come to be seen as an outdated irrelevance in a clinical context. When asked if he 'recognises the existence of spiritual interests' in his patients, Lydgate is unwilling to address the subject, only noting that 'those words are apt to cover different meanings to different minds'.[400] In recognising that the personal, subjective nature of spirituality was at odds with the medical move towards empirically verifiable and notionally objective things, Eliot exposed the tension that continues to hamper the provision of spiritual care in the contemporary NHS. Many clinicians still see spirituality as a 'meaningless term' or refuse to accept that it is a 'valid concept' within a healthcare context,[401] because of its vague, subjective qualities. Yet what I have discovered is that integrating the arts into spiritual care can facilitate care practices and resources that accommodate 'different meanings' and 'different minds'. Indeed, Eliot's use of literary fiction to probe the relationship between 'spiritual interests' and medicine is itself an illustration of the value of the arts as an alternative means of accessing and exploring the spiritual domain.

As Eliot noticed, spiritual care 'depends on the person'.[402] Yet she also foresaw that the project of modern medicine necessitated 'the reducing of the particular to the general', in order to clear the way for 'scientific achievement'.[403] I believe we can meet the 'spiritual need for a lost sense of humanity' that emerged during the 'roaring age of Evidence-Based-Medicine'.

While in this work I have limited myself to exploring the care of cancer patients, the implications of my research could be productively applied, I believe, to other conditions. Across society, the number of patients requiring spiritual support is rapidly growing in an ageing population affected by long COVID, increasing rates of cancer diagnosis and chronic illness, and the social care crisis. Popular artworks with a wide appeal can, I believe, become invaluable resources in efforts to meet this urgent, increasing, and much broader need for spiritual care. In this regard, specialists in other areas of healthcare, such as dementia care and care for the homeless, have suggested to me that my approach to arts-based spiritual care could be valuable for many, if not all, NHS patients.

POSTSCRIPT

The last section of Ewan's notebook is labelled 'Conclusion', and comprises the three paragraphs transcribed below:

My hope is that this book has been read as an expression of gratitude. When I set out to write, my intention was to convey my indebtedness to other people. The meaning that I have found in my illness and dying has been borrowed from others: authors, creators, artists, fellow patients, friends and family. It was only by turning outwards and opening myself to the creativity and generosity of these people that I have learned to tell my story.

I also hope that telling this story will help other patients in need of encouragement or inspiration to remain open to a range of stories. I believe that when it comes to interpreting and responding to disease, we are surrounded by rich resources. Embedded in a culture of spiritual searching, we do not have to look far to find a vast range of imaginative perspectives on our mortality.

As the tumour invades new areas of my brain, its influence and impact spreading, I can feel my energy slipping away. My capacity for profound, precise thought feels like it is a long-lost memory. The range of things that I can do is shrinking. And in this state of deepening disability and limitations, I can only engage with literature and art that is clear and comforting, treating the reader or viewer with charity and compassion.

ACKNOWLEDGEMENTS

I would like to thank Maggie's Cancer Care centres (Maggie's), and the Northumberland Cancer Support Group (NCSG) for their generosity in supporting my research. I would also like to thank the patients that use these charities for the courage and kindness they showed in participating in my research projects and sharing stories that were moving, enlightening and inspiring.

I would like to thank George Corbett for his consistently superb supervision and pastoral support, and John Swinton for his invaluable assistance.

Finally, I would like to thank my endlessly encouraging and generally fantastic family (Jane, Chris, Alfie, Laura and Lads) and my wise and wonderful wife, Karlee, for the countless ways that they have found to help me through difficult moments and allow me to thrive. I love and cherish you all, and I couldn't have wished for a better support team!

This work was supported by a SGSAH AHRC Doctoral Training Partnership for Scotland with funding by the Scottish Graduate School for Arts & Humanities, the UKRI Arts and Humanities Research Council, and the Scottish Funding Council.

Resources
Ewan's complete thesis, 'From Beaune to *Breaking Bad*: Using the Arts to Meet Cancer Patients' Need and Desire for Spiritual Care' is available online: https://doi.org/10.17630/sta/243

For a pdf of the *Maggie's Fiction Library Guide* go to: https://theoartistry.org/maggies-fiction-library/

Publishing
Ewan's family would like to thank the team at DLT for everything they have done to bring this work to publication.

ENDNOTES

Part I, Chapter 2: Borrowed Stories
1. Frank, *Wounded Storyteller*, 3.
2. *Ibid.*, 2.
3. *Ibid.*, 2.
4. *Ibid.*, 5.
5. Frankl, *Man's Search for Meaning*, 86-89.
6. *Ibid.*, 94.
7. *Ibid.*, 109.
8. Frank, *Wounded Storyteller*, 197.
9. *Ibid.*, 197-200.
10. *Ibid.*, 197-98.
11. *Ibid.*, 200.
12. *Ibid.*, 200.
13. Will Schwalbe, *The End of Your Life Book Club* (London: John Murray Press, 2012), 7.
14. *Ibid.*, 8.
15. A good example of this is Sara Liyanage's article, 'Ticking Off Breast Cancer,' *Making Maggie's*, November 1, 2019, 21.
16. In Ewan's notebook, the word here transcribed as 'spirit' is not completely clear.

Part II, Chapter 1: Rethinking Spiritual Care
17. Wilfred McSherry, 'Enhancing and Advancing Spiritual Care in Nursing and Midwifery Practice,' *Nursing Standard* 35, no. 10 (2020): 65-68.
18. For more on the 'spiritual heritage' of nursing, see Tony Walter,

'Developments in Spiritual Care of the Dying,' *Religion* 26 (1996): 353-63; Dorothy C. H. Lee and Inge B. Corliss, 'Spirituality and Hospice Care,' *Death Studies* 12, no. 2 (1988): 101-10.

[19] Daniel E. Hall, Harold G. König, and Keith G. Meador, 'Conceptualizing 'Religion': How Language Shapes and Constrains Knowledge in the Study of Religion and Health,' *Perspectives in Biology and Medicine* 47, no. 3 (2004): 386-401 (387).

[20] John Swinton, 'Spirituality in Healthcare,' *Journal for the Study of Spirituality* 4, no. 2 (2014): 162-73.

[21] See, for instance, Richard Egan, Anna Graham-DeMello, Sande Ramage and Barry Keane, 'Spiritual Care: What Do Cancer Patients and their Family Members Want? A Co-design Project,' *Journal for the Study of Spirituality*, 8:2 (2018), 142-159; Anja Visser, Bert Garssen, and Ad Vingerhoets, 'Spirituality and Well-being in Cancer Patients: A Review,' *Psychooncology*, 19 (2009): 565-72; Alan B. Astrow, Ann Wexler, Kenneth Texeira, M. Kai He, and Daniel P. Sulmasy, 'Is Failure to Meet Spiritual Needs Associated with Cancer Patients' Perceptions of Quality of Care?,' *Journal of Clinical Oncology*, 25 (2007): 5753-57.

[22] Nessa Coyle and Betty R. Ferrell, *The Nature of Suffering and the Goals of Nursing* (Oxford: Oxford University Press, 2008), 3.

[23] See Rina Arya, 'Spirituality and Contemporary Art,' *Oxford Research Encyclopaedias: Religion* (Published online 31st August 2016), https://doi.org/10.1093/acrefore/9780199340378.013.209; Kutter Callaway and Barry Taylor, *The Aesthetics of Atheism: Theology and Imagination in Contemporary Culture* (Minneapolis: Fortress Press, 2019); Jeremy Begbie, *Redeeming Transcendence in the Arts: Bearing Witness to the Triune God* (London: SCM Press, 2018).

[24] Gordon Lynch, 'The Role of Popular Music in the Construction of Alternative Spiritual Identities and Ideologies,' *Journal for the Scientific Study of Religion* 45, no. 4: 481-84. Lynch also notes that popular music is often overlooked in research investigating how media can play a role in 'the formation of religious identity and meaning'. Whilst this clearly merits further study, the thematic methodology for spiritual care tested in this project, and my lack of knowledge or expertise in the field of popular music, mean this is not the place to undertake that research. However, I briefly allude to the

ENDNOTES

capacity for a piece of popular music to initiate and enrich shared meaning-making in Chapter 5 (p.135).

[25] There is still 'much debate' concerning forms of art therapy involving patients in 'visual art-making'. For more on this, see Chapter 1, p. 25, and also Kristina Geue, Heide Goetze, Marianne Buttstaedt, Evelyn Kleinert, Diana Richter, and Susanne Singer, 'An Overview of Art Therapy Interventions for Cancer Patients and the Results of Research,' *Complementary Therapies in Medicine* 18 (2010): 160-70, and Xiao-Han Jiang, Xi-Jie Chen, Qin-Qin Xie, Yong-Shen Feng, Shi Chen, Jun-Sheng Peng, 'Effects of Art Therapy in Cancer Care: A Systematic Review and Meta-Analysis,' *European Journal of Cancer Care* 29, no. 5 (Published Online June 15, 2020), https://doi.org/10.1111/ecc.13277.

Part II, Chapter 2: Spiritual Care and the Arts

[26] Sulmasy, *Rebirth*, 70.

[27] Bakker, 'Spirituality,' 33-34.

[28] Swinton et al., 'Moving Inward,' 645.

[29] Fitch and Bartlett, 'Patient Perspectives,' 117.

[30] Julie A. Ponto et al., 'Stories of Breast Cancer through Art,' *Oncology Nursing Forum* 30, no. 6 (2003): 1007-13. Research into cancer patients' responses to photographic art in wards also showed that patients 'valued' the art and found that certain works conveyed 'optimism and safety', or an important 'symbolic meaning'. See Hazel Hanson et al., 'Preferences for Photographic Art for Hospitalised Patients with Cancer,' *Oncology Nursing Society* 40, no. 4 (July 2013), 338-42.

[31] Kevin E. Bras, 'Meditation as Spiritual Intervention', in *Spirituality and Meaning in Health Care: A Dutch Contribution to an Ongoing Discussion*, ed. Jake Bouwer (Leuven: Peeters, 2008), 112-13, 140.

[32] Weaver, *Theology of Suffering*, 105-111.

[33] Michael Baum, preface to *Something Understood: Art Therapy in Cancer Care*, ed. Camilla Connell (London: Wrexham Publications, 1998), 8.

[34] Reasons for cancer patients rejecting, or ending prematurely, art-therapy interventions include: 'a lack of interest in art, a sense of incompetence ("I cannot paint") or illness-related complications'. See Geue et al., 'An Overview of Art Therapy Interventions'.

[35] Jiang et al., 'Effects of Art Therapy in Cancer Care'.
[36] Groves and Klauser, *American Book of Living and Dying*, 205
[37] Connell, *Something Understood*, 14.
[38] Many of the artworks listed here were included in the 'Maggie's Fiction Library' resource that I produced for Maggie's Cancer Care Centres. For more information see pages 32-40 of this chapter, and to view a PDF of the *Maggie's Fiction Library Guide*, see https://theoartistry.org/maggies-fiction-library/
[39] These collaborations also involved a four-month internship with the Northumberland Cancer Support Group, in which I explored how artworks could be used to facilitate and generate discussion of spiritual concerns and foster a sense of community for shielding patients during the first COVID-19 lockdown. Having been forced to adapt the plans for the internship in response to COVID restrictions, I designed – in collaboration with the support group committee and specialist therapists – new ways of providing spiritual support to members when meeting in-person was impossible. This included running an online 'NCSG Reading Group', in which members of the support group were encouraged to read novels or watch television series that would form the basis of group discussions. The popular novels and television series selected were intended to be an accessible, engaging means of opening up themes such as time, uncertainty and community that were especially relevant for members of a cancer support group during the pandemic. Unfortunately, there was not time to secure the necessary ethical approval to gather data from the online Reading Group. This was particularly frustrating because evidence from the group revealed that structuring virtual communities around reflection on, and discussion of, popular artworks can sustain and enrich interactions between members of cancer support groups. Commenting on the Reading Group, the NCSG chairperson said: 'this was very successful. Many members responded positively, sharing their reactions to the novels or series, and connecting these to their own experiences of cancer, as well as relating the novels or series to their experiences of NCSG and the reasons they value the group'. See Frances Davies, 'Internship/Artist-in-Residence Programme Host Organisation Feedback Form,' *SGSAH*, July 27, 2020.

ENDNOTES

Part II, Chapter 3: Cancer, Time and Fiction

[40] Nicola Christie, 'How Did *The Fault in Our Stars* Become a Bestseller and Hollywood Hit Movie,' *The Independent*, June 12, 2014, https://www.independent.co.uk/arts-entertainment/books/features/how-did-fault-our-stars-tough-talking-book-about-two-teenagers-dying-cancer-become-bestseller-and-hollywood-hit-movie-9530575.html.

[41] Margaret Talbot, 'The Teen Whisperer,' *New Yorker*, June 2, 2014, https://www.newyorker.com/magazine/2014/06/09/the-teen-whisperer.

[42] Emily T. Katz, 'John Green Explains How a Failed Attempt at Divinity School Inspired 'The Fault in Our Stars',' *HuffPost*, March 25, 2015, https://www.huffingtonpost.co.uk/entry/john-green.

[43] John Green, 'Interview with John Green,' Goodreads, December 4, 2012. https://www.goodreads.com/interviews/show/828John_Green.

[44] Katz, 'John Green Explains'.

[45] See, for instance, Alan Lewis's claim that this culture has come to be defined by 'timidity and negation' in its dealings with death and disease, and by a collective 'loss of meaning, hope, and creativity (*Cross and Resurrection*, 341-48). This fatalistic perspective is shared by Timothy Keller, who argues in his own theology of cancer that contemporary Western culture 'gives people almost no tools for dealing with tragedy' (*Walking with God*, 15-16).

[46] To date, there has been little or no academic scholarship reflecting on *The Fault in Our Stars* as a fictional exploration of spiritual themes relating to cancer. One notable exception is Trudelle Thomas's article 'The Spiritual Quest amid Loneliness, Depression, and Disability: Reflections on The Fault in Our Stars by John Green,' *Religious Education* 113, no. 1 (2018): 73-83.

[47] Anwar Deeb, 'Moments of Infinite Joy within a Limited Time: The Concept of Time in John Green's The Fault in Our Stars,' *International Journal of English and Literature* 7 (2016): 112-14.

[48] *Ibid.*, 114.

[49] Whilst in a Soviet prison camp, Solzhenitsyn was told he was in urgent need of surgery to treat a tumour, then made to wait two weeks until the operation. During this delay, 'he felt his tumour swell, distending his stomach almost hourly'. Donald M. Thomas,

Alexander Solzhenitsyn: A Century in his Life (London: Little, Brown and Company, 1988), 223

50 Lewis, *Between Cross and Resurrection*, 412-13.

51 This process is exactly what the author Will Schwalbe describes in *The End of Your Life Book Club* (London: Two Roads, 2012). Schwalbe explains how discussing fictional characters from novels with his mother, while she was receiving treatment for terminal cancer, enabled them to broach sensitive subjects relating to cancer and time, such as when it would be 'time to stop' treatment (175).

52 See Anna Obergfell Kirkman, Jane A Hartsock, and Alexia M Torke, 'How The Fault in Our Stars Illuminates Four Themes of the Adolescent End of Life Narrative,' *Medical Humanities* 45 (2019): 240. Kirkman, Hartsock and Torke focus on four themes directly relevant to adolescent cancer patients: (1) the paradox of emerging autonomy and limited lifespan, (2) intensity of emotions (3) the desire to have significant experiences on an accelerated timeline and (4) preferences around legacy and memory-making. In this section I focus on cancer patients' spiritual needs, showing how Green's novel also illuminates four themes relating to time that have a broader relevance and are likely to affect all cancer patients.

53 Deeb, 'Moments of Infinite Joy,' 116.

54 Tiesinga, 'Spirituality of the Professional in Health Care,' in *Spirituality and Meaning in Health Care: A Dutch Contribution to an Ongoing Discussion*, ed. Jake Bouwer (Leuven: Peeters, 2008), 54.

55 Gordon, *Dying and Creating*, 49.

56 Kübler-Ross, *Death and Dying*, 207-9.

57 Bain et al., 'The Role of Spirituality in the Early Stages of Breast Cancer,' 647.

58 See Chapter One, 28.

59 Solzhenitsyn, *Cancer Ward*, 268.

60 For a similarly affecting fictional scene dramatising the impact of 'lost time' caused by a cancer diagnosis, see series 2 of *Cold Feet: Series 8*, in which Jenny Gifford (played by Fay Ripley) hears her son discussing plans for an eighteenth birthday party whilst concealing her fear that she will not be alive to take part in the festivities. See *Cold Feet*, season 8, episode 2, directed by Rebecca Gatward, written by Mike Bullen, aired January 14, 2019, https://www.britbox.co.uk/series/S8_43341.

ENDNOTES

61 Solzhenitsyn, *Cancer Ward*, 166.
62 *Ibid.*, 168.
63 Lewis, *Between Cross and Resurrection*, 93.
64 Rudd and Worlding, 'The Management of People with Advanced Head and Neck Cancers,' 240.
65 Lewis, *Between Cross and Resurrection*, 404-13.
66 *Ibid.*, 413. See also Schwalbe's description of hospitals as 'interruption factories', in *The End of Your Life Book Club*, 49.
67 Hatice Guz, Bilge Gursel and Nilgun Ozbek, 'Religious and Spiritual Practices among Patients with Cancer,' *Journal of Religion and Health* 51, no. 3 (September 2012): 769.
68 Solzhenitsyn, *Cancer Ward*, 54-5.
69 Kirkman, Hartsock, and Torke, 'How The Fault in Our Stars Illuminates,' 243.
70 Green, *The Fault in Our Stars*, 158.
71 For another example of a poignant evocation of the 'cruel' routines of cancer treatment, see Patrick Ness's novel *A Monster Calls* (London: Walker Books, 2015), in which a young boy gradually becomes habituated to the process of watching his mother made ill by cycles of chemotherapy: 'It was always the second and third days after treatment that were the worst... It had become almost normal' (45-47).
72 *Ibid.*, 197.
73 Connell, *Something Understood*, 81.
74 Lewis, *Between Cross and Resurrection*, 409.
75 Solzhenitsyn, *Cancer Ward*, 324.
76 A hugely popular television series that recently captured this perspective is *The Crown: Series 4*, in which Princess Margaret (played by Helena Bonham Carter) struggles to find 'meaning' in life, or to 'fill her time', as she undergoes treatment for incurable breast cancer. See *The Crown: Series 4*, directed by, Paul Whittington, Julian Jarrold, Jessica Hobbs, and Benjamin Caron, written by Peter Morgan, aired November 15, 2020, Netflix, https://www.netflix.com/watch/80215488? trackId=14277283.
77 Green, *The Fault in Our Stars*, 82.
78 *Ibid.*, 116.
79 For another fascinating literary insight into a patient's experiences of waiting in a hospital ward, see Jean Dominique Bauby's depiction

of his time in hospital following an accident that left him paralysed, in *The Diving Bell and the Butterfly* (London: HarperCollins, 2002): 'A mysterious paradox: time, motionless here, gallops out there' (p. 109).

80 Swinton, 'Beyond Clarity,' 234.

81 *Horizon*, 'We need to talk about death,' produced by Rob Liddel, featuring Kevin Fong, aired January 23, 2019, BBC iPlayer, https://www.bbc.co.uk/programmes/p06yc17v.

82 Green, *The Fault in Our Stars*, 13. Intriguingly, the fictitious novel *An Imperial Affliction* was based on David Foster-Wallace's *Infinite Jest*, which itself is a 'transposition' of Dostoevsky's *The Brothers Karamazov*. Wallace promoted Dostoevsky as a 'model' for fiction writers striving against modern manifestations of the nihilism that Dostoevsky's novels ridiculed, and suggested that contemporary authors can produce 'holograms' of these novels, following Dostoevsky in juxtaposing unflinching portrayals of human vulnerability and powerful, persuasive hopefulness (see Timothy Jacobs, 'The Brothers Incandenza: Translating Ideology in Fyodor Dostoevsky's *The Brothers Karamazov* and David Foster Wallace's *Infinite Jest*,' *Texas Studies in Literature and Language* 49, no. 3 (2007): 265-292). Wallace himself took up this challenge in *Infinite Jest*, then Green re-mediated Dostoevsky's 'hopeful perspective' in *The Fault in Our Stars*, adopting the 'model' Dostoevsky's fiction provides and applying it to the challenging spiritual landscape of the new millennium. For more on this, see my article entitled 'John Green's *The Fault in Our Stars*: A Novel Contribution to 'The Field of Thinking About Suffering,'' *Journal of Religion and Popular Culture* (published online May 3rd, 2022), https://doi.org/10.3138/jrpc.2021-0014.

83 Green, *The Fault in Our Stars*, 39.

84 Alison Milbank, 'Apologetics and the Imagination,' in *Imaginative Apologetics: Theology, Philosophy and the Catholic Tradition*, ed. Andrew Davison (London: SCM Press, 2011), 39-40.

85 Janet M. Soskice, *Metaphor and Religious Language* (Oxford: Oxford University Press, 1987), 120-33.

86 Solzhenitsyn, *Cancer Ward*, 518-27.

87 Ibid., 518-22.

88 David Brown, *Discipleship and Imagination: Christian Tradition and Truth* (Oxford: Oxford University Press, 2004), 74.

ENDNOTES

89 Stoddard, *The Hospice Movement*, 209.

90 Green, *The Fault in Our Stars*, 149. There are interesting parallels between Gus's response to his terminal diagnosis and the Mitja Okorn film *Life in a Year*, in which a seventeen-year-old boy sets out to give his girlfriend 'a life in a year' after she is diagnosed with terminal cancer. A sense of the inventive, naïve defiance of the strictures of time is identifiable in Okorn's film, which explores questions of quality and quantity of life with the same youthful, imaginative exuberance identifiable in Green's novel. See *Life in a Year*, directed by Mitja Okorn (2020; Culver City: Columbia Pictures), Amazon Prime, https://www.amazon.co.uk/Life-Year-Cara-Delevingne/dp/B08XYBSYR8.

91 See, for instance, Gordon, *Dying and Creating*, 49.

92 Another bestselling novel that examines the disparities between 'clock time' and a personal 'inner time' exposed by disease, is Audrey Niffenegger's novel *The Time Traveller's Wife* (London: Vintage Books, 2005). This fictional tale of time-travel, illness and romance investigates 'how it feels to be living outside of the time constraints most humans are subject to', and to 'live, fully present, in the world' in moments when 'Time is nothing'. (pp. 445, 504). A participant in the Fiction Library trial, identifying as a professional Maggie's psychologist, commented that *The Time Traveller's Wife* 'brings to the forefront my therapeutic work in terms of helping people accept the uncertainty in their lives and to live in the moment'. Highlighting the potential relevance of the novel to a cancer patient seeking a more constructive relationship to time, the participant suggested this fictional narrative would be a useful resource for those they were caring for: 'If working with a client regarding accepting uncertainty I could suggest *The Time Traveller's Wife*… [as] a nice way in to explore topics that may need a light touch to begin with' (FL: 7, 13).

93 *Ibid.*, 272-73.

94 Aleksandr Solzhenitsyn, *The Gulag Archipelago*, trans. Thomas P. Whitney (London: Collins and Harvill Press, 1974), 484.

95 John Green, Epigraph in *The Fault in Our Stars*. There are interesting parallels here with contemporary theological fiction which challenges inflexible, linear conceptions of time, such as Eugene Vodolazkin's novel *Laurus*, which describes a sacred environment in

which '[t]ime no longer moves forward but goes around in circles', exploring the idea of time as a 'spiral' and 'open figure', whilst also contrasting this with less imaginative notions of temporality within the secular sphere. See Vodolazkin, *Laurus*, trans. Lisa Hadyn (London: Bloomsbury, 2015). For more on the imaginative treatment of time in *Laurus*, see my article "Time is Not All Powerful': the Eschatological Vision in Eugene Vodolazkin's *Laurus*', *Literature and Theology* (Published Online 7th September 2021), https://doi.org/10.1093/litthe/frab022.

[96] *Ibid.*, 11-13.

[97] Swinton, 'Beyond Clarity', 234.

[98] *Ibid.*, 358.

[99] Michel Aucoutrier, 'Solzhenitsyn's Art,' in *Solzhenitsyn: A Collection of Critical Essays*, ed. Katherine Feuer (New Jersey: Prentice Hall, 1976), 29.

[100] Weaver, *Theology of Suffering and Death*, 128. Cancer patients see being present 'in the moment' as an important aspect of spiritual coping during illness. See Margaret I. Fitch and Ruth Bartlett, 'Patient Perspectives about Spirituality and Spiritual Care,' *The Asia Pacific Journal of Oncology* 6, no. 2 (2019): 113.

[101] Aucoutrier, 'Solzhenitsyn's Art,' 29-30.

[102] Lucy Kalanithi, Epilogue, in *When Breath Becomes Air*, by Paul Kalanithi (London: Vintage, 2017), 218.

[103] Green, *The Fault in Our Stars*, 191-98.

[104] *Ibid.*, 233.

[105] Richard Bauckham, 'Time, Eternity and the Arts,' in *Art, Imagination and Christian Hope*, eds. Trevor Hart, Gavin Hopps and Jeremy Begbie (Burlington: Ashgate, 2012), 7-19. Frankl offers Tolstoy's novella *The Death of Ivan Ilyich* as an example of work of fiction that reveals how lives tragically transformed by illness can be punctuated by moments of 'infinite meaning'. See *Man's Search for Meaning*, 129-31.

[106] *Green, The Fault in Our Stars*, 116.

[107] Mitch Albom's autobiographical *Tuesdays with Morrie* traces a comparable shift in perspective, as the eponymous Morrie, who is dying of cancer, transforms Albom's attitude towards time by revealing how a tragically truncated life can become qualitatively rich: 'I envied the quality of Morrie's life even as I lamented its

diminishing supply'. See Albom, *Tuesdays with Morrie* (London: Sphere, 2013), 34-43.

108 Christopher Swift, 'Speaking of the Same Things Differently,' in *Spirituality in Health Care Contexts*, ed. Sarah Orchard (London: Jessica Kingsley Publishers, 2001), 99.

109 See, for instance, the debates over the withdrawal of the drug Avastin for cancer patients: Jeremey Laurence, 'The Cost of NHS Health Care: Deciding Who Lives and Who Dies,' *The Independent*, March 9, 2015, https://www.independent.co.uk/life-style/health-and-families/features/cost-nhs-health-care-deciding-who-lives-and-who-dies-10096784.html. Or the refusal of NICE to approve the drug Kadcyla for the treatment of breast cancer: Jennifer Rigby, 'Why the NHS Thinks a Healthy Year of Life is Worth £20,000,' *Channel 4 News*, April 23, 2014, https://www.channel4.com/news/drugs-life-breast-cancer-nice-20-000-a-year-of-life-nhs.

110 Groves and Klauser, *The American Book of Living and Dying*, 196-97.

111 Green, *The Fault in Our Stars*, 260.

112 An interesting parallel in popular culture to Hazel's discovery of a 'forever within the numbered days' can be found in the Richard Curtis film *About Time*. In a complex plot involving an inherited capacity to time travel, the death of Tim Lake's father from cancer transforms his own perspective on time, leading him to 'try to live every day as if I've deliberately come back to this one day to enjoy it: as if it was the full final day of my extraordinary life' – in other words, to try to treat every day as a 'little infinity'. See *About Time*, directed by Richard Curtis (2013; Universal City: Universal Pictures), Amazon Prime, https://www.amazon.co.uk/About-Time-Domnhall-Gleeson/dp/B00IK9O8QU.

113 For more on *The Time Traveller's Wife*, see footnote 284 in this chapter.

114 Green's evocation of a 'forever' amid transient life is consonant with Oliver Sacks' profound theological response to his terminal cancer, which was grounded in '[t]he peace of the Sabbath, of a stopped world, a time outside time'. As he died, Sacks found himself drawn to 'little emblems of eternity' symbolic of this atemporal seventh day. See Sacks, *Gratitude* (London: Picador, 2016), 44-45. Green's novel could help cancer patients to discover how a short, painful life

might be replete with the 'emblems of eternity' that Sacks discovered.

[115] For more on authorial authority in *The Fault in Our Stars* see Tara Moore, '"Death of the Author" in the Literature Classroom and John Green's The Fault in Our Stars,' *Children's Literature in Education* (May 2021): 1-13.

[116] Green is renowned for his willingness to engage with readers, answering their questions and listening to their unique interpretations of his novels, including many young cancer patients who have related to *The Fault in Our Stars*. See Margaret Talbot, 'The Teen Whisperer,' *New Yorker*, June 2, 2014, https://www.newyorker.com/magazine/2014/06/09/the-teen-whisperer.

[117] Describing the development of Van Houten's character, Green says that he 'wanted to think about the relationship between the people who create the things we love and the things themselves', and 'our instinct to conflate the two even though the people are often at least as flawed as we are'. See Anon., 'Interview with John Green,' *Goodreads*, December 4, 2012, https://www.goodreads.com/interviews/show/828.John_Green.

[118] Green, *The Fault in Our Stars*, 68.

[119] Kaila Hale-Stern, 'Pop Culture Is Obsessed with Time-Loops, Time Travel, and Alternate Worlds,' *The Mary Sue*, February 25, 2019, https://www.themarysue.com/we-are-obsessed-with-time/.

[120] See Alison Flood, 'Sales of Mind, Body, Spirit Books Boom in UK amid 'Mindfulness Mega-Trend',' *The Guardian*, July 31, 2017, https://www.theguardian.com/books/2017/jul/31/sales-of-mind-body-spirit-books-boom-in-uk-amid-mindfulness-mega-trend.

[121] John Miedema, 'Back to Books: The Joy of Slow Reading,' *The Guardian*, October 13, 2018, https://www.theguardian.com/lifeandstyle/2018/oct/13/joy-of-slow-reading-books.

Part II, Chapter 4: Cancer, Paradox and Breaking Bad

[122] See, for instance, Keller, *Walking with God*, 15-17.

[123] Craig Simpson, 'Hurtling toward Death,' in *Breaking Bad and Philosophy*, eds. David R. Koepsell and Robert Arp (Chicago: Open Court, 2012), 63. For more examples of this 'TV landscape', see footnote 358.

[124] James Monaco, *How to Read a Film* (Oxford: Oxford University Press, 2000), 506.

ENDNOTES

[125] Grace Chu-Hui-Lin Chi, 'The Role of Hope in Patients with Cancer,' *Oncology Nursing Forum* 34, no. 2 (April 2007): 415.

[126] Frankl, *Man's Search for Meaning*, 92.

[127] See Chapter 1, 4-5.

[128] The sources from my qualitative research referenced in this chapter are Transcript 1, Maggie's Dundee, November 4, 2019; and Transcript 5, held via Microsoft Teams, January 22, 2021. These anonymised transcripts will be referenced in the main text as (TR: page number). This chapter also makes use of the transcript collating the anonymised questionnaires from the Fiction Library trial, which will be referenced in the main text as (FL: page number). For more information on these sources, see the 'Sources' section in the front matter of my thesis.

[129] Restivo, *Breaking Bad and Cinematic Television*, 4.

[130] Brian Gibson, 'Romancing the Ice: The Problematic Poetry of Breaking Bad,' *Critical Studies in Television* 13, no. 4 (2014): 406.

[131] Restivo, *Breaking Bad and Cinematic Television*, 4.

[132] *Ibid.*, 26.

[133] Hilmes et al., 'Rethinking Television,' 27.

[134] *Ibid.*, 37.

[135] *Ibid.*, 44-5.

[136] Robert K. Johnston, *Reel Spirituality: Theology and Film in Dialogue* (London: Baker Academic, 2006), 20.

[137] See, for instance, 'Welcome to the Breaking Bad Wiki,' *Breaking Bad Wiki*, accessed August 2, 2021, https://breakingbad.fandom.com/wiki/Breaking_Bad_Wiki.

[138] Eric San Juan, *Breaking Down Breaking Bad* (Create Space Independent Publishing Platform, 2013), 48-9.

[139] See, for instance, San Juan, *Breaking Down Breaking Bad*; David R. Koepsell and Robert Arp, eds., *Breaking Bad and Philosophy* (Chicago: Open Court, 2012).

[140] See @Breaking Bad, Twitter, accessed August 3, 2021, https://twitter.com/breakingbad.

[141] See 'Breaking Bad', Facebook, accessed August 3, 2021, https://www.facebook.com/BreakingBad/.

[142] Pamela Brown, *Facing Cancer Together* (Minneapolis, Augsburg Press, 1999), 13.

[143] San Juan, *Breaking Down Breaking Bad*, 11.

[144] Edgar N. Jackson, *Counselling the Dying* (London: SCM, 1981), 1-2.
[145] Mark Porter, 'How to Talk About Cancer,' *The Times*, January 29, 2019, 36. See also Susan Sontag's discussion of the 'military flavour' of the language used to describe cancer treatment, in *Illness as Metaphor* (New York: Farrar, Strauss and Giroux, 1988), 6-8.
[146] Nell Dunn, *Cancer Tales* (Charlbury: Amber Lane Press, 2002), 26.
[147] Christie Watson, *The Language of Kindness: A Nurse's Story* (London: Chatto and Windus, 2019), 261.
[148] *Horizon*, 'We Need to Talk About Death,' produced by Rob Liddel, featuring Kevin Fong, aired January 23, 2019, BBC iPlayer, https://www.bbc.co.uk/programmes/p06yc17v.
[149] Chi, 'The role of hope,' 415.
[150] Bob Cleland, 'I Was Given Hope,' in *Strength from our Lives*, ed. Liza Wolfe (Glasgow: Spectra Print, 2007), 28.
[151] Gibson, 'Romancing,' 409-10.
[152] *Breaking Bad*, created by Vince Gilligan, aired January 20, 2008, AMC, Netflix, https://www.netflix.com/title/70143836 [following the convention within Television Studies, references to *Breaking Bad* from this point are given in the main text as (series: episode)].
[153] David R. Koepsell and Robert Arp, 'A Fine Meth We've Gotten Into,' in *Breaking Bad and Philosophy*, eds. Koepsell and Arp (Chicago: Open Court, 2012), viii.
[154] San Juan, *Breaking Down Breaking Bad*, 60-1.
[155] Lisa Kadonaga, 'You're Supposed to Be a Scientist,' in *Breaking Bad and Philosophy*, eds. David R. Koepsell and Robert Arp (Chicago: Open Court, 2012), 187.
[156] Simpson, 'Hurtling toward Death,' 61.
[157] Groves and Klauser, *American Book of Living and Dying*, 64-5.
[158] Darryl J. Murphy, 'Heisenberg's Uncertain Confession,' in *Breaking Bad and Philosophy*, eds. David R. Koepsell and Robert Arp (Chicago: Open Court, 2012), 16.
[159] Porter, 'How to Talk About Cancer,' 36.
[160] Christina Faull, *The Handbook of Palliative Care*, 3rd ed. (Hoboken, NJ: Wiley-Blackwell, 2012), 1.
[161] Kubler-Ross, *Death and Dying*, xv-xi.
[162] Bakker, 'Spirituality and Meaning,' 42.
[163] Powe, 'Cancer Fatalism,' 135.

ENDNOTES

[164] Guz et al., 'Religious and Spiritual Practices,' 769.
[165] Sara Liyanage, 'Ticking Off Breast Cancer,' *Making Maggie's*, November 1, 2019, 21.
[166] Hinton, *Dying*, 95.
[167] Following the convention within Television Studies, references to *Breaking Bad* from this point will be given in the main text as (series number, episode number).
[168] Marsh and Ortiz, introduction to *Theology and Film*, 14. For another insightful fictional exploration of the anxiety-inducing effects of a cancer ward, see Garth Stein's novel *The Art of Racing in the Rain* (London: Harper Collins, 2009). Narrated by a dog, Enzo, who can smell the 'chemical release' of emotions such as 'Tension. Fear. Anxiety', the novel thus offers the reader access to the private, concealed feelings of Enzo's owner, Eve. Whilst Eve undergoes treatment for cancer, Enzo reveals the psychological, spiritual impact of this ordeal for Eve: 'She was so afraid of doctors and hospitals. She was afraid she might go in and they would never let her out' (77-81).
[169] For more on the use of fictional scenes of doctor-patient interactions from television series to encourage conversation and promote understanding between patients and caregivers, see my article "Talk to Me Like I Was a Person You Loved': Including Patients' Perspectives in Cinemeducation', *Intima* (Published online March 1, 2021), https://www.theintima.org/perspectives-in-cinemeducation-by-ewan-bowlby. I describe how, listening to patients' commentaries on scenes of doctor-patient interactions, healthcare professionals became aware of how patients 'see things differently', alerting them to crucial perspectival factors that influence patients' interpretations of their encounters with clinicians. Studying the discussions of these scenes in focus groups reveals how audio-visual narratives can support this collaborative process of discovery, affording a shared space in which mutual understanding can flourish.
[170] Simpson, 'Hurtling toward Death,' 60.
[171] Maclaren, 'Presence,' 20.
[172] Brandon L. Mick, 'Redemption's Stage,' in *Cancer and Theology*, eds. Jake Bouma and Erik Ullestad (Des Moines: Elbow Co., 2014), 77.
[173] Frankl, *Man's Search for Meaning*, 131.

[174] Gordon, *Dying and Creating*, 12.

[175] Weaver, *The Theology of Suffering and Death*, 92.

[176] Connell, *Something Understood*, 36.

[177] Swinton, 'Spirituality in Healthcare', 169-70.

[178] Cassidy, *Sharing the Darkness*, 76.

[179] *Ibid.*, 5-11.

[180] Gordon, *Dying and Creating*, 165.

[181] Nelson, *Human Medicine*, 24.

[182] Gibson, 'Romancing,' 407.

[183] *Ibid.*, 410-11.

[184] James Parker, 'Til Meth Do Us Part: Who is Going to Die at the End of *Breaking Bad*,' *The Atlantic*, July/August 2013, 44-6.

[185] Another notable example of a fictional character who displays an innovative and potentially inspiring form of 'creative resignation' to terminal cancer is Lisa Johnson (played by Kerri Godliman), in the dark television comedy *After Life*. Whilst she is dying of cancer, Lisa has recorded 'a little guide to life without me' for her husband Tony (Ricky Gervais). Her creative legacy becomes a source of meaning amidst the nihilistic grief that threatens to consume Tony after her death. See *After Life*, created and directed by Ricky Gervais, aired March 8, 2019, Derek Productions Limited, Netflix, https://www.netflix.com/title/80998491.

[186] An audio-visual artwork that could draw families into a discussion of different forms of 'creative resignation', affording compelling, inspiring examples, is the Disney-Pixar animated film *Coco*, directed by Lee Edward Unkrich and Adrian Molina (2017; Emeryville, CA: Pixar Animation Studios), Amazon Prime, https://www.amazon.co.uk/Coco-Theatrical-Version-Anthony-Gonzalez/dp/B0792CPZDW. Set during the Mexican Day of the Dead holiday, *Coco* offers families and younger viewers colourful, alluring visions of the traditional rituals, symbolism, and mythology used to commemorate and celebrate loved ones during the *Día de Muertos*, as well as luring viewers into the vibrant, lively 'Land of the Dead'. *Coco* thus presents imagery and concepts that frame death as a natural and even joyful step beyond the quotidian world.

[187] Paul MacInnes, '*Breaking Bad*: 10 years on, TV is still in Walter White's shadow,' *The Guardian*, November 8, 2018, https://www.theguardian.com/tv-and-radio/2018/jan/20/breaking-bad-10-

years-on-tv-is-still-in-walter-whites-shadow.
188 DuBose, 'Meaning of Meaninglessness,' 293.
189 Restivo, *Breaking Bad and Cinematic Television*, 11.
190 P. Brown, *Facing Cancer Together*, 68.
191 For a charming, child-friendly fictional study of the interrelationship of life and death, see E. B. White's novel *Charlotte's Web* (London: Penguin, 2003). The sage, compassionate spider, Charlotte, helps the frantic and naïve young pig, Wilbur, to reconcile himself to her death through illustrating how a death can lead into new life. With her last energy, Charlotte gives birth to a host of infant spiders, and weaves an intricate web as part of an ingenious plan to save Wilbur's life. Fascinatingly, one of the participants in the Fiction Library trial commented that 'the pig's [Wilbur's] denial even though Charlotte was clearly dying' was an aspect of the story that felt 'helpful' and 'relevant' to their personal situation (FL: 3).
192 Stephen Glass, 'Better Than Human,' in *Breaking Bad and Philosophy*, eds. David R. Koepsell and Robert Arp (Chicago: Open Court, 2012), 93.
193 Gordon, *Dying and Creating*, 14-16.
194 Dan Miori, 'Was Skyler's Intervention Ethical?', in David R Koepsell and Robert Arp, eds. *Breaking Bad and Philosophy* (Chicago: Open Court, 2012), 28-33.
195 Bain et al., 'The Role of Spirituality,' 646
196 See Todd's description of herself and another patient awaiting radiotherapy: '[w]e're such *memento mori*, he and I. Both of us with mouths sand-paper dry'. *Radiation Diaries*, 125.
197 Swinton, 'Spirituality in Healthcare,' 170-71.
198 Brown, *Facing Cancer Together*, 15.
199 *Ibid.*, 643.
200 Robin Kirkpatrick, introduction to *The Inferno*, Dante Alighieri, trans. Kirkpatrick (London: Penguin, 2005), ixxv.
201 Louise France, 'Victoria Derbyshire: My Breast Cancer Diary,' *The Times*, September 9, 2017, https://www.thetimes.co.uk/article/victoria-derbyshire-my-breast-cancer-diary-thshx5gc7.
202 Liyanage, 'Ticking Off Breast Cancer,' 21.
203 P. Brown, *Op. cit.*, 12-13.
204 Cunningham, 'I Needed to Accept,' 124.
205 This is the same scene discussed earlier in this chapter (74-5). There

were two distinct forms of response to this scene in the focus group: on the one hand, several participants related to the sense of shock and disorientation it conveyed, whilst others were prompted by the scene to reflect on and discuss the importance of dependence and family support (see above).

[206] Johnston, *Reel Spirituality*, 154-55.

[207] Another fictional narrative that can afford insight for a cancer patient struggling to embrace interdependence is Iain Banks's novel *The Quarry* (London: Hachette, 2013). Kit, who has autism, is caring for his father, Guy, who is dying of cancer. Described from the perspective of Kit, as first-person narrator, the unusual relationship between these two protagonists mingles anger and resentment with love and loyalty, reflecting the complexity of father-son relations whilst also revealing how meaning and 'wholeness' can emerge amidst the conflict and confusion that cancer can cause.

[208] See Kirkpatrick, introduction to *The Inferno*, lxxv. For more on Dante's use of negative imagery in the *Inferno* see, for instance, John Freccero, 'Bestial Sign and Bread of Angels: Inferno xxxii and xxxiii,' in *Dante: The Poetics of Conversion* (Cambridge, Mass.: Harvard University Press, 1986), 152-66.

[209] Robin Kirkpatrick, *Dante's Inferno: Difficult and Dead Poetry* (Cambridge: Cambridge University Press, 2008), 6.

[210] Kirkpatrick, commentary on *The Inferno*, 445-47.

[211] For a more detailed exploration of the idea of Walter White as a revealing 'silhouette' of alternative choices that he did not make, see my article 'Drugs, Death, Denial and Cancer Care: Using *Breaking Bad* in the Spiritual Care of Cancer Patients,' *Critical Studies in Television* 15, no. 3 (2020): 223-38. Using the theological concept of a 'silhouette of goodness', and Jung's theory of the ego-life and True Self, as analytical tools, this article suggests that symbolic moments in Walt's descent into chaotic criminality could help caregivers to meet the 'need for symbols' in cancer care.

[212] Monaco, *How to Read a Film*, 514.

[213] Telford, 'Through a Glass Darkly,' 16.

[214] Johnston, *Reel Spirualty*, 14.

[215] Kirkpatrick, commentary on *The Inferno*, 447.

[216] For example, Stephen Sutton raising £5 million for cancer charities [Rebecca Gillie, 'Stephen Sutton: £5 Million Legacy of

ENDNOTES

Inspirational Cancer Teen,' *Huffington Post*, September 16, 2014, https://www.huffingtonpost.co.uk/2014/09/16/stephen-sutton-5-million-legacy-of-inspirational-cancer-teen_n_7322530.html]; the remarkable work of journalist and presenter Rachel Bland [Catherine Pepinster, 'Rachael Bland had Guts. But She Did Not 'Fight a Battle' Against Cancer,' *The Guardian*, September 6, 2018, https://www.theguardian.com/commentisfree/2018/sep/06/rachael-bland-battle-cancer-bbc-presenter]; or Lynn Joseph climbing Everest weeks after cancer treatment [Nilufer Atik, 'I Climbed Thousands of Feet up Everest during Cancer Treatment,' *iNews*, May 10, 2019, https://inews.co.uk/news/teacher-climbed-up-everest-whilst-in-the-middle-of-cancer-treatment-289840].

[217] Ernest Becker, *The Denial of Death* (London: Free Press 1997), ix.

[218] Arguably, the iconography created by the audio-visual imagery in *Breaking Bad* can meet the 'need for symbols' in contemporary cancer care. For more on this, see my article 'Drugs, Death, Denial and Cancer Care: Using *Breaking Bad* in the Spiritual Care of Cancer Patients,' *Critical Studies in Television* 15, no. 3 (2020): 223-38.

[219] Keller, *Walking with God*, 55.

[220] See, for instance, Liddel, *Horizon*, 'We Need to Talk About Death.'; *Grayson Perry: Rites of Passage*, series 1, episode 1, 'Death,' directed by Neil Crombie, featuring Grayson Perry, aired August 23, 2018, Swan Films, All4, https://www.channel4.com/programmes/grayson-perry-rites-of-passage.

[221] See, for instance, Deborah James, Laura Mahon and Rachel Bland, 'You, Me and the Big C,' first aired March 7, 2018, BBC iPlayer, https://www.bbc.co.uk/programmes/p0608649/episodes/guide; D. S. Moss, 'The Adventures of Memento Mori,' first aired February 17, 2021, Apple Podcasts, https://podcasts.apple.com/us/podcast/the-adventures-of-memento-mori/id1061189831?mt=2.

[222] See, for instance, the moving story of grief, enchantment, and spiritual searching *Onward*, directed by Dan Scanlon (2020; Burbank, CA: Walt Disney Studios), Amazon Prime, https://www.amazon.co.uk/Onward-Plus-Bonus-Content-Officer/dp/B08617YZ8W; or Molina and Unkrich's hugely popular children's animation *Coco* [see footnote 194].

[223] The 'Departure Longue' in Lewisham is an instillation aimed at tackling taboos surrounding death and dying. See Joanna Moorhead, 'Welcome to the Departure Lounge. Destination: Death,' *The Guardian*, May 5, 2019, https://www.theguardian.com/lifeandstyle/2019/may/05/welcome-to-the-deaprture-lounge-destination-death.

Part II, Chapter 5: The Bucket List: Levity, Laughter and Living with Cancer

[224] The term 'cancer comedy' has come to be used in popular discourse to denote a comedy combining humour and an exploration of aspects of living with cancer. See, for instance, Cath Clarke, 'Running Naked Review – Feelgood Cancer Comedy with Teen Pranks,' review of *Running Naked*, *The Guardian*, February 1st, 2021, https://www.theguardian.com/film/2021/feb/01/running-naked-review-feelgood-cancer-comedy-with-teen-pranks.

[225] *The Bucket List*, directed by Rob Reiner (2007; Burbank, California: Warner Brothers), Amazon Prime, https://www.amazon.co.uk/Bucket-List-Jack-Nicholson/dp/B00EU76F5S [references to *The Bucket List* from this point are given as (minutes) in the main text].

[226] There are some discussions of *The Bucket List* in academic scholarship, although these are usually in somewhat esoteric fields. See, for example, Thomas Turnell-Read, '"What's on Your Bucket List?': Tourism, Identity and Imperative Experiential Discourse,' *Annals of Tourism Research* (November 2017): 58-66; Rizky Abdul Rachman, 'Existentialism in the Character Study: Carter and Cole in *The Bucket List* Movie,' *Lantern* 2, no. 2 (2013): 1-5.

[227] McCreaddie and Wiggins observe that, in healthcare contexts, 'humour, somewhat paradoxically, is something that is generally not taken seriously'. See May McCreaddie and Sally Wiggins, 'The Purpose and Function of Humour in Health, Health Care and Nursing: A Narrative Review,' *Journal of Advanced Nursing* 61, no. 6 (March 2008): 591.

[228] May McCreaddie and Sheila Payne, 'Humour in Health-Care Interactions: A Risk Worth Taking,' *Health Expectations* 17, no. 3 (January 2012): 332-34.

[229] The sources from my qualitative research referenced in this chapter are transcripts of the recordings from the focus group trials, and are as

follows: Transcript 2, held in person at Maggie's Dundee, November 9, 2019; Transcript 3, held via Microsoft Teams, December 8, 2020; and Transcript 4, held via Microsoft Teams, November 4, 2020. These anonymised transcripts will be referenced in the main text as (Transcript: page number). For more information on these sources, see the front matter of this thesis.

[230] David Browne, 'Films, Movies, Meanings,' in *Explorations in Theology and Film: An Introduction*, eds. Clive Marsh and Gaye Ortiz (Oxford: Blackwell, 1997), 9.

[231] Kyle Smith, 'Two Good Men,' review of *The Bucket List*, *New York Post*, December 25, 2007, https://nypost.com/2007/12/25/two-good-men/.

[232] Richard Corliss, 'Death Myths,' review of *The Bucket List* and *Savages*, *Time*, December 26, 2007, http://content.time.com/time/arts/article/0,8599,1698307,00.html.

[233] Deborah Ross, 'Count Me Out,' review of *The Bucket List*, *The Spectator*, February 13, 2008, https://www.spectator.co.uk/article/count-me-out.

[234] Ebert, 'O Death.'

[235] Corliss, 'Death Myths.'

[236] Deacy, introduction to *Faith in Film*, vi.

[237] Pamela Grace, *The Religious Film: Christianity and the Hagiopic* (New Jersey: Wiley, 2009), 13.

[238] See Zsófia Demjén, 'Laughing at Cancer: Humour, Empowerment, Solidarity and Coping Online,' *Journal of Pragmatics* 101 (2016): 18. Demjén notes that '[a]t the 2015 Edinburgh Festival Fringe Beth Vyse, Alastair Barrie and Adam Hills were among those who based their comedy routines on their own or their partner's cancer experiences'. This chapter references several other recent examples of 'cancer comedy' within popular culture, including: a) films: *50/50*, directed by Jonathan Levine (2011; Santa Monica, California: Lionsgate), Netflix, https://www.netflix.com/title/70202141; *Funny People*, directed by Judd Apatow (2009; Universal City, California: Universal Pictures), Amazon Prime, https://www.amazon.co.uk/Funny-People-Adam-Sandler/dp/B001954AYA; *Running Naked*, directed by Victor Buhler (2021; Seattle: Amazon Prime Video), Amazon Prime, https://www.amazon.co.uk/Running-Naked-Tamzin-Merchant/dp/B08SMRR3WZ; b) television series:

Catastrophe, season 1, episode 1, directed by Ben Taylor, written by Sharon Horgan and Rob Delaney, aired January 19, 2015, Channel 4, https://www.channel4.com/programmes/catastrophe/on-demand/58083-001; *Orange is the New Black*, season 2, episode 8, 'Appropriately Sized Pots,' directed by Daisy von Scherler Mayer, written by Alex Regnery and Hartley Voss, aired June 6, 2014, Netflix, https://www.netflix.com/watch/70296535; c) novels: Iain Banks, *The Quarry* (London: Little, Brown, 2013); d) pathography: Adam Blain, *Pear Shaped: The Funniest Book So Far this Year About Brain Cancer* (Seattle, Washington: Amazon Publishing, 2015); and e) stand-up comedy: Billy Connolly, 'Colonoscopy,' YouTube, February 24, 2008, https://www.youtube.com/watch?v=BBMsPNI6EZE.

[239] McCreaddie and Wiggins note that we must understand how humour is used in the 'non-sterile, complex and dynamic environments in which we actually live' to integrate humour into patient care successfully. See 'The Purpose and Function of Humour,' 591-92.

[240] Rob Reiner, interview by David Poland, DP/30: The Oral History of Hollywood, YouTube, July 21, 2014, https://www.youtube.com/watch?v=NZ7z1K5FkzA.

[241] Christie and Moore, 'Impact of Humour,' 211.

[242] Rahner, *Man at Play*, 29.

[243] Hopps, 'Comedy,' 244.

[244] Slavoj Žižek, *Did Somebody Say Totalitarianism?: Five Interventions in the (Mis)use of a Notion* (London: Verso, 2001), 68, quoted in Hopps, 'Comedy,' 244. Hopps also notes that humour thereby can paradoxically 'communicate by advertising a failure of communication', enabling the expression of things which might otherwise seem unutterably awful or incomprehensible (244).

[245] Nathan Scott, *The Broken Centre* (London: Yale University Press, 1966), 89-90.

[246] Hyers, *The Comic Vision*, 122.

[247] J. M. Cohen, introduction to *Don Quixote*, Cervantes, trans. Cohen (Harmondsworth: Penguin, 1950), 16. This carefree disregard for the limitations of the world as it is fits neatly with the Christian proleptic imagination, which anticipates the future realisation of a new, divine game on earth. Early Christian scholar Origen's declaration that 'the truly wise man is like a child that smiles and plays' reveals that this theological defence of the playful comic 'protest' derives from the

scriptural concept of the 'foolishness' of God in Christ (1 Corinthians 20 etc.), which calls into question all worldly wisdom. See Origen, *In Mattheum*, quoted in Rahner, *Man at Play*, 37.
[248] Rahner, *Man at Play*, 36.
[249] Hyers, *The Comic Vision*, 36.
[250] Hopps, 239-40.
[251] Paul McGhee, 'Rx: Laughter,' *RN* 61, no. 7 (1998): 50-53.
[252] Kalanithi, *When Breath Becomes Air*, 88-89.
[253] Watson, *Language of Kindness*, 268.
[254] Hopps, 'Comedy,' 245.
[255] The importance of play and distraction on a cancer ward is also explored in the Netflix dramedy *Orange is the New Black*. Rosa Cisneros (discussed in Chapter 1, p. 12), befriends a young boy who is undergoing chemotherapy alongside her and, drawing on her experience as bank robber, constructs an elaborate game involving a 'heist' on the ward to entertain and distract her companion. The warmth and comedy captured in their imaginative play affords glimpses of how a cancer ward can become associated with more than just repetitious suffering. See *Orange is the New Black*, season 2, episode 8, 'Appropriately Sized Pots,' directed by Daisy von Scherler Mayer, written by Alex Regnery & Hartley Voss, aired June 6, 2014, Netflix, https://www.netflix.com/watch/70296535.
[256] Indeed, the film affords a fun, fictional illustration of the findings of studies suggesting that men with cancer can use humour to 'reduce tension and share a sense of solidarity with others'. See Allison Chapple and Sue Ziebland, 'The Role of Humor for Men with Testicular Cancer,' *Qualitative Health Research* 14, no. 8 (2004): 1123.
[257] Mark Porter, 'How to Talk About Cancer.' *The Times*, January 29, 2019.
[258] Kester Brewin, 'A Theopraxis of Cancer,' in *Cancer and Theology*, ed. Jake Bouma and Erik Ullestad (Des Moines: Elbow Co, 2014), 41-42.
[259] Rahner, *Man at Play*, 29.
[260] Carter's deadpan delivery and sarcasm are reminiscent of Billy Connolly's stand-up routine in which he expertly exploits the strangeness and discomfort of a colonoscopy for comic effect, demystifying and reframing a process that might otherwise seem

daunting. See Billy Connolly, 'Colonoscopy,' YouTube, February 24, 2008, https://www.youtube.com/watch?v=BBMsPNI6EZE.

261 The tangible significance of the shared humour here is highlighted in real clinical trials, as patients who used joking and banter displayed an improved pain threshold and immune response, as well as 'elevations in natural killer cell activity' when reacting to tumours. See Christie and Moore, 'Impact of Humour,' 211.

262 Barbara Fraley, and Arthur Aron, 'The Effect of a Shared Humorous Experience on Closeness in Initial Encounter,' *Personal Relationships* 11, no. 1 (March 2004): 61-78.

263 Lucy Kalanithi, epilogue to *When Breath Becomes Air*, 213-14.

264 Watson relates how her father's deathbed became a place to 'cry and laugh' as her father died with 'humour, dignity and a complete lack of fear'. See *Language of Kindness*, 271.

265 Caroline Bainbridge, 'Television as Psychical Object: Mad Men and the Value of Psychoanalysis for Television Scholarship,' *Critical Studies in Television* 14, no. 3 (August 2019): 299-302.

266 Piper 'That's Life,' 89. Frankl explains this phenomenon by suggesting that becoming 'absorbed in play' can connect patients to the 'humanness of man [and woman]', enriching their Search for Meaning, in *Man's Search for Meaning*, 84-85.

267 Hyers, *The Comic Vision*, 122.

268 Johnston, *Reel Spirituality*, 23.

269 Cole's refusal to take seriously his prognosis is indicative of the control he has reassumed over the course of his life with cancer, revealing the power his comic vision has granted him. This form of power was also revealed in the real-life story of a comedian who 'made up songs' and 'cracked jokes' during awake brain surgery to 'break the ice'. She was able to use humour to change the 'atmosphere' of the operating theatre into a scenario 'like being in a café with your friends', transforming a traumatic procedure into an uplifting occasion and amusing story. See Lynsey Hope, 'Comedian Cracks Jokes from her Stand-up Routine while Having a Brain Tumour Removed in 9-hour Operation,' *The Sun*, August 25, 2018, https://www.thesun.co.uk/news/7096237/comedian-cracks-jokes-from-her-stand-up-routine-while-having-a-brain-tumour-removed-in-9-hour-operation/.

270 This inventive use of humour to transform how a cancer diagnosis

ENDNOTES

is perceived is redolent of the scene in the Channel 4 sitcom *Catastrophe*, in which an oncologist's attempts to convey a diagnosis of 'pre-cancer' descend into farcical misunderstanding. As Sharon, the protagonist (played by comedian Sharon Horgan), tries to make sense of this diagnosis – 'so just a half-cancer then' – her playful wisecracking softens the emotional blow of the encounter, alerting viewers to an alternative to the passive role of the anxious, confused patient receiving shocking news. See *Catastrophe*, season 1, episode 1, directed by Ben Taylor, written by Sharon Horgan and Rob Delaney, aired January 19, 2015, Channel 4, https://www.channel4.com/programmes/catastrophe/on-demand/58083-001.

[271] Melissa P. Masterson, Elizabeth Slivjak, Greta Jankauskaite, William Breitbart, Hayley Pessin, Elizabeth Schofield, Jason Holland, and Wendy G. Lichtentha. 'Beyond the Bucket List: Unfinished Business among Advanced Cancer Patients,' *Psycho-Oncology* 27, no. 11 (November 2018): 2573-80.

[272] Moyra Sidell. 'Treatment or Tender Loving Care,' in *Care Matters: Concepts, Practice and Research in Health and Social Care*, ed. Ann Brechin, Jan Walmsley, Jeanne Samson Katz, and Sheila M. Peace (London: Sage Publications, 1998), 96-106.

[273] Margaret Fitch and Ruth Bartlett, 'Patient Perspectives about Spirituality and Spiritual Care,' *Asia-Pacific Journal of Oncology Nursing* 6, no. 2 (April-June 2019): 117.

[274] Hopps, 'Comedy,' 243-47.

[275] *Ibid.*, 239-40.

[276] Robin Kirkpatrick, commentary on *Paradiso*, Dante Alighieri, trans. and ed. Robin Kirkpatrick (London: Penguin, 2007), 470.

[277] Branney et al., 'Masculinities,' 2057.

[278] A study investigating spirituality and boredom in cancer patients suggested that these concepts are crucial to our understanding of quality of life in advanced cancer patients. See Alice Inman, Kenneth L. Kirsh, and Steven D. Passik, 'A Pilot Study to Examine the Relationship between Boredom and Spirituality in Cancer Patients,' *Palliative and Supportive Care* 1, no. 2 (2003): 143-51.

[279] For instance, *The Fault in Our Stars* contains the passage relating to flying and 'living longer' analysed in chapter 2, in which Gus uses the physics of flight to capture and express his developing

understanding of a more personal, open sense of time; *Ways to Live Forever* by Sally Nicholls (London: Marion Lloyd Books, 2008) describes how flying in an airship allows a young boy living with cancer to see his situation from a 'very different angle' (164); Elizabeth Berg's novel *Talk Before Sleep* (New York: Ballantine Books, 2006) suggests that seeing the 'toylike' cars and 'beauty' of the world 'down there' viewed from an aeroplane can bring 'truth' to someone affected by cancer (115).

Part II, Chapter 6: Cancer, Emotion and Sentimentality

[280] As there is – as I will show – no agreed definition of what constitutes 'sentimental' art, I will use the word here to refer to formal features of these popular artworks which have either been described as, or would likely be considered to be 'sentimental', on the basis of the exhaustive list of aesthetic and ethical qualities deemed sentimental provided by Marcia Eaton, in 'Laughing at the Death of Little Nell: Sentimental Art and Sentimental People,' *American Philosophical Quarterly* 26, no. 4 (1989): 269-82. It is also worth noting that both *Cold Feet* and *Talk Before Sleep* have been described as 'sentimental' (see below, footnotes 200-204, 216, 220), so that their specific features of narrative, imagery, dialogue etc. are also likely to be described as such.

[281] The sources from my qualitative research referenced in this chapter are Transcript 7, held via Microsoft Teams, March 9, 2021; and Transcript 6, held via Microsoft Teams, November 10, 2020. These anonymised transcripts will be referenced in the main text as (Transcript: page number). This chapter also makes use of the transcript collating the anonymised questionnaires from the Fiction Library trial, which will be referenced in the main text as (Fiction Library: page number). For more information on these sources, see the front matter of this thesis.

[282] Stoddard, *Hospice Movement*, 3.

[283] Chi, 'Role of Hope,' 449.

[284] Bruce Charlton, 'Life Before Health: Against the Sentimentalisation of Medicine,' in *Faking It: The Sentimentalisation of Modern Society*, ed. Digby Anderson and Peter Mullen (London: Social Affairs Unit, 1998), 21-23.

[285] Mary Deshazer, *Fractured Borders* (Michigan: University of

Michigan Press, 2006), 170-71.
[286] Sontag, *Illness as Metaphor*, 3.
[287] Deshazer, *Fractured Borders*, 135.
[288] Mark Jefferson, 'What is Wrong with Sentimentality,' *Mind* 92, no. 368 (1983): 519-21.
[289] An excellent example of this confusion is Digby Anderson and Peter Mullen's edited volume of essays *Faking It: The Sentimentalisation of Modern Society* (London: Social Affairs Unit, 1998), which uses the idea of sentimentality to justify polemics against everything from the overcooking of a roast dinner (see Anderson, 'Self-indulgence, Childishness and Puritanism', 147-61), to the loss of 'discipline and obedience' in schools (see Bruce Cooper and Dennis O'Keeffe, 'Sweetness and Light in Schools', 53-81).
[290] Jefferson, 'What is Wrong with Sentimentality,' 524. Similarly, Mary Midgley argues that being sentimental is 'misrepresenting the world in order to indulge our feelings', in 'Brutality and Sentimentality,' *Philosophy* 54, no. 209 (July 1979): 385). In this view, any emotion evoked through the 'dishonest distortion of reality' is objectionable, regardless of the nature of that emotion (Jefferson, 'What is Wrong with Sentimentality,' 523.)
[291] Gregory Woolfe, 'Editorial Statement: The Painter of Lite,' *Image* 34 (2002): 5, quoted in Begbie, 'Beauty,' 54.
[292] Stoddard, *Hospice Movement*, 5.
[293] Solomon, *Defense of Sentimentality*, 3.
[294] *Ibid.*, 5.
[295] Jefferson, 'What is Wrong with Sentimentality,' 525. Although, far from being a 'syrupy' confection cut off from reality, the death of Little Nell was a 'a culturally specific response to a particular set of circumstances' – sentimental fiction 'perfectly attuned to the emotional needs of [the] age' conveying a 'commonplace of consolation' amongst bereaved parents. See Richard Walsh, 'Why We Wept for Little Nell: Character and Emotional Involvement,' *Narrative* 5, no. 3 (October 1997): 308. I also offer a more detailed defence of this scene in my article highlighting the significance on context in considering matters of 'sentimentality': "French Endings': Christianity, Sentimentality and the Arts in the Context of Covid,' *International Journal for The Study of the Christian Church* 22, no.2 (June 2022): 111-23.

296 Marsh, *Cinema and Sentiment*, 31.
297 See, for instance, Saul Friedlander, *Reflections on Nazism: Essays on Kitsch and Death* (New York: Harper and Row, 1989); Peter Wicke, 'Sentimentality and High Pathos: Popular Music in Fascist Germany,' *Popular Music* 5 (1985): 149-58.
298 Stoddard, *Hospice Movement*, 29.
299 Oscar Wilde, Letter to Lord Alfred Douglas, in *The Letters of Oscar Wilde*, ed. Rupert Hart-Davis (London: Rupert Hart-Davis, 1962), 501, quoted in Begbie, 'Beauty,' 53.
300 Solomon, *Defense of Sentimentality*, 1-2.
301 Jefferson, 'What is Wrong with Sentimentality,' 32.
302 Begbie, 'Beauty,' 46-47.
303 William Stringfellow, *A Keeper of the Word: Selected Writings of William Stringfellow*, ed. Bill W. Kelleron, (Grand Rapids: Eerdmans, 1994), 62. There is a tendency in the Western world to search for a spiritual 'silver lining' when confronting suffering or loss (McLaren, 'Presence,' 21), which lies behind the deeply unsatisfactory and 'pseudo-spiritual phrases frequently offered to cancer patients' (Bouma and Ullestad, introduction to *Cancer and Theology*, xii).
304 Begbie, 'Beauty,' 48-49.
305 *Ibid.*, 52.
306 Begbie, 'Beauty,' 52-54.
307 Begbie, *Redeeming Transcendence*, 86.
308 Begbie, 'Beauty,' 51.
309 Milan Kundera, *The Unbearable Lightness of Being* (New York: Harper and Row, 1989), 251, quoted in Begbie, 'Beauty,' 50.
310 Begbie, 'Beauty,' 54.
311 *Ibid.*, 56-57, 63-64.
312 Begbie, 'Beauty,' 48.
313 *Ibid.*, 61-63.
314 *Ibid.*, 47-49. This touches on a point made in Gregory Syler's theology of cancer, which warns against the 'theological mistake' of trivialising the impact of cancer by 'layering the suffering with Hallmark platitudes', when 'pain and suffering' should always be treated as 'profound and truly powerful realities'. See Syler, 'On Pain, Suffering and Cancer,' in *Cancer and Theology*, eds. Jake Bouma and Erik Ullestad (Des Moines: Elbow Co, 2014), 97-99.
315 Begbie, 'Beauty,' 60.

ENDNOTES

[316] *Ibid.*, 60.
[317] Fyodor Dostoevsky, *The Brothers Karamazov*, trans. Constance Garnett (Harmondsworth: Penguin, 1958), 267 [references to *The Brothers Karamazov* from this point given as page numbers in the main text].
[318] Ivan's words do indeed resonate with those of real people affected by cancer, such as the mother of a child dying of leukaemia: 'when I get to heaven, there's going to be some serious conversation between me and God'. See Ferrell and Coyle, *The Nature of Suffering*, 9.
[319] Bell, *Sentimentalism*, 205-6.
[320] Jefferson, 'What is Wrong with Sentimentality,' 520.
[321] Robert C. Solomon, 'On Kitsch and Sentimentality,' quoted in David Morgan, *Visual Piety: History and Theory of Popular Religious Images* (California: University of California Press, 1999), 30.
[322] Marsh, *Cinema and Sentiment*, 31.
[323] Jane Tompkins, *Sensational Designs: The Cultural Work of American Fiction 1790-1860* (Oxford: Oxford University Press, 1986), 21.
[324] Bell, *Sentimentalism*, 160.
[325] Fraser Watts, 'Self-Conscious Emotions, Religion and Theology,' in *Issues in Science and Theology: Do Emotions Shape the World?*, eds. Dirk Evers et al. (Zurich: Springer International Publishing, 2016), 209.
[326] Otis, *Banned Emotions*, 3.
[327] Marianne Noble, *The Masochistic Pleasures of Sentimental Literature* (Princeton: Princeton University Press, 2000), 8.
[328] Marsh, *Cinema and Sentiment*, 70.
[329] 648 Ibid., 69.
[330] Dolores Morehead, quoted in Hope, *Help Me Live*, 158.
[331] Otis, *Banned Emotions*, 1.
[332] Wendy Harper, quoted in Julie K. Silver, *What Helped Me Get Through: Cancer Survivors Share Wisdom and Hope* (Atlanta, GA: American Cancer Society, 2008), 29. Elsewhere, I have written about the 'dangers of denial' for cancer patients (see Ch. 3, especially), so it is worth clarifying why I am suggesting that it can also be a positive thing in these circumstances. The key distinction is between the forms of 'temporary but needed denial' described here (brief respite from emotional and physical pain), and the kind of violent, all-consuming, ceaseless denial practised by Walter White in *Breaking Bad*.

[333] Hinton, *Dying*, 105
[334] *Ibid.*, 105.
[335] Halina Irving, quoted in Hope, *Help Me Live*, 48.
[336] Nicholas Wolterstoff, *Art in Action: Toward a Christian Aesthetic* (Grand Rapids: Eerdmans, 1980), 147.
[337] Charlton, 'Life Before Health,' 21.
[338] Otis, *Banned Emotions*, 8.
[339] Spiegel, M., quoted in Hope, *Op. cit.*, 136.
[340] Otis, *Banned Emotions*, 3.
[341] Susan Kerr, 'Positive from Negative', in Wolfe, *Strength from Our Lives*, 149.
[342] Hope, *Help Me Live*, 96.
[343] Hope, *Help Me Live*, 138.
[344] Begbie, 'Beauty,' 48.
[345] Maggie's Barts, 'Annette's Story – Will Writing,' Facebook, November 28, 2019, https://www.facebook.com/watch/?v=530718957479979.
[346] Another patient explains how there were times when she wanted simple emotional reassurance from her oncologist, instead of direct, clinical realism: 'I wish my doctor had just held my hand and said, ''I know this is awful, but you will be okay'' (Silver, *What Helped Me*, 84). This might resemble what an anti-sentimentalist would refer to as emotion 'divorced from the intellect' (Begbie, 'Beauty,' 53), but the experiences of cancer patients show that these simple gestures can 'mean everything'.
[347] Solomon, *Defense of Sentimentality*, 11.
[348] Marsh, *Cinema and Sentiment*, 11.
[349] *Ibid.*, 11.
[350] Kirkus, 'Talk Before Sleep,' review of *Talk Before Sleep*, Book Reviews, March 1, 1994, https://www.kirkusreviews.com/book-reviews/elizabeth-berg/talk-before-sleep/.
[351] Deshazer, *Fractured Borders*, 138, 171.
[352] *Ibid.*, 147.
[353] Walsh, 'Why We Wept,' 308.
[354] *Ibid.*, 155
[355] GoodReads, 'Talk Before Sleep,' Community Reviews, accessed March 29, 2020, https://www.goodreads.com/book/show/127390.Talk_Before_Sleep.

ENDNOTES

356 Deshazer, *Fractured Borders*, 155.

357 Elizabeth Berg, foreword to *Talk Before Sleep* (London: Arrow Books, 2004). [References to *Talk Before Sleep* after this point are given in the main body of the text as (page numbers).]

358 Book Reporter, 'Talk Before Sleep,' review of *Talk Before Sleep*, May 24, 2011, https://www.bookreporter.com/reviews/talk-before-sleep.

359 Anonymous, quoted in Deshazer, *Fractured Borders*, 155.

360 Anonymous, quoted in Deshazer, *Fractured Borders*, 155.

361 Jasper Rees, 'Cold Feet, Series 8, ITV, Review – Mortality Lite,' review of *Cold Feet: Series 8*, *The Arts Desk*, January 15, 2019, https://www.theartsdesk.com/tv/cold-feet-series-8-itv-review-mortality-lite.

362 Sean O'Grady, 'Cold Feet Review – Less than the Sum of its Parts', *The Independent: Arts and Entertainment* (13th January 2020).

363 Thomas Sutcliffe, 'Cold Feet: The End of the Affair,' *The Independent*, March 13, 2003, https://www.independent.co.uk/news/media/cold-feet-the-end-of-the-affair-122482.html.

364 Fay Ripley, 'I End up Hugging People on Trains,' interview by Gloria Dunn, *The I*, January 11, 2020, 51.

365 *Ibid.*, 51.

366 This connection was also apparent in the public response to *Cold Feet: Series 9*, in which Jenny's cancer storyline continues. In my article 'All Around, though Often Invisible': Using *Cold Feet: Series 9* in the Spiritual Care of Cancer Survivors', *The Postgraduate Journal of Medical Humanities* 7 (2021): 52-76, I describe how this television drama sheds light on the specific challenges long-term cancer survivors face following discharge. The series remained an especially apposite case-study because there is evidence that people affected by the issues raised continued to find value in Jenny's storyline. Series 9 'struck a chord' with survivors and analysing its spiritual affordances reveals why this was the case. The challenge to the 'restitution narrative' it presents, allied to an exploration of the complexities of relationships after treatment, and of the difficulties of finding an alternative illness narrative, affords material to borrow that could help survivors to find their voice and navigate new, unfamiliar challenges. Therefore, *Cold Feet: Series 9* is also an illustration of the capacity for accessible, fictional narratives to be used to engage

with an area of experience that contemporary healthcare, and society as a whole, struggles to address.

[367] Sarah Hughes, 'Cold Feet Has Finally Become Must-watch TV ... 22 Years after it Started,' *The Guardian*, February 18, 2019, https://www.theguardian.com/tv-and-radio/2019/feb/18/cold-feet-finally-must-watch-tv-series-eight.

[368] Sue Long, 'Cold Feet Storyline Strikes a Chord,' Maggie's Online Community: Blog, February 12, 2020.

[369] Bell, *Sentimentalism*, 206.

[370] *Ibid.*, 206. For a novel that could draw younger readers into a comparable exercise of 'emotional discrimination', see Paterson's *Bride to Terabithia*. Jess, the young protagonist of the story, feels frustrated by the 'red-eyed adults' struggling to come to terms with the death of Jess's best friend, Leslie. Rather than acknowledging or expressing his own feelings of loss, Jess's interior monologue is full of scorn for Leslie's father, who cries 'like someone in an old mushy movie' (156-68). Like Dostoevsky's Kolya, Jess becomes a parody of the ideal of male 'strength' and anti-sentimentality, exposing the societal inclination towards emotional suppression in the face of emotional pain.

[371] *Cold Feet: Series 8*, directed by Rebecca Gatward and John Hardwick, aired January 14, 2019, ITV, Britbox, https://www.britbox.co.uk/series/S8_43341 [following the convention within Television Studies, references to *Cold Feet: Series 8* from this point are given in the main text as (series: episode)].

[372] This thought-provoking exploration of emotional reticence is redolent of the suppression and silence found in the cancer 'tear-jerker' classic, *Stepmom*, directed by Chris Columbus (1998; Culver City, CA: Sony Pictures Releasing), Netflix, https://www.netflix.com/title/18171073. In this film combining romance, discord and terminal cancer, Susan Sarandon plays a terminally ill mother struggling to accept her ex-husband's new lover, who will become her children's stepmother. Having shown Jackie (Sarandon) undergo an MRI scan and receive a terrifying prognosis, her face a picture of shock and incomprehension, the film cuts straight to a meeting between Jackie and her ex-husband, Luke, who tells Jackie that he is planning to marry his girlfriend, Isabel (Julia Roberts). Luke, unaware of the powerful feelings of shock and fear that Jackie is experiencing,

discusses plans for the future and for their children: 'we are still their parents for the next hundred years'. Yet the audience, aware of Jackie's 'emotional truth', can sense the pain behind her tearful eyes and shaking voice (81-84mins). Rather than telling Luke her devastating news, as she had planned, Jackie choses to hide her emotional turmoil, affording a poignant illustration of the isolation such suppression can cause.

373 Walsh, 'Why We Wept,' 318. Katherine Erskine's novel *Mockingbird* (London: Usborne Publishing, 2012) also affords a space for this form of discursive self-examination. Narrated by Caitlin, who has Asperger's, Erskine allows a neurodiverse perspective to influence how the emotions surrounding a tragic high school shooting are perceived. Caitlin is aware that emotions are 'not one of [her] strengths', yet her attempts to understand the diverse forms of suppressed, disguised grief she witnesses are paradoxically revealing and insightful (53-57).

374 Greg Garrett, a theologian writing about his experiences of cancer, captures the value of this form of affordance. After receiving the 'sterile emotion-less diagnosis of an overwhelmed doctor', he describes how he watched the film *Stepmom* (1998), in which a lead character is dying of cancer, and 'cried like a four-year-old with a bloody stained knee'. See Garrett, 'Death and Resurrection,' in *Cancer and Theology*, eds. Jake Bouma and Erik Ullestad (Des Moines: Elbow Co, 2014), 36-37. For further discussion of the Chris Columbus film *Stepmom*, see footnote 157.

375 Dolores Morehead, quoted in Hope, *Help Me Live*, 158.

376 Richard Carnevale, review of *Cold Feet Series 8: Episode 3*, indieLondon, January 29, 2019.

377 Mary Gallagher, 'My Pain: Cold Feet's Fay Ripley Reveals She Was Crying Real Tears over Dying Father When She Filmed Jenny's Devastating Cancer Diagnosis,' *The Sun*, January 28, 2019, https://www.thesun.co.uk/tvandshowbiz/8296830/cold-feet-fay-ripley-father-jenny-cancer/.

378 The genre of 'tearjerker' films about cancer has become a popular feature of contemporary fictional explorations of living with cancer. Notable examples include: *Miss You Already*, directed by Catherine Hardwick (2015; Toronto: Entertainment One), Amazon prime, https://www.amazon.co.uk/Miss-You-Already-Toni-Collette/dp/B08V8DL3FL, a film about cancer and female companionship

that 'isn't shy about going for filmgoers' tear ducts' (see 'Critic's Consensus', Rotten Tomatoes, accessed September 29, 2021, https://www.rottentomatoes.com/m/miss_you_already); and *A Walk to Remember*, directed by Adam Shankman (2002; Burbank, CA: Warner Brothers), Google Play, https://play.google.com/store/movies/details/Nur_mit_Dir?id=oGjMzilcn9o&gl=US, based on Nicholas Spark's sentimental novel about young love, faith and cancer. It seems likely that the enduring popularity of this genre of film is, in part, due to their capacity to give viewers 'permission' to release feelings caused by real-life experiences of illness or tragedy.

[379] Marsh, *Cinema and Sentiment*, 31, 69.

[380] When she has Ann observe that they 'even saw a few men wiping their eyes' following *Sophie's Choice* it becomes clear she has set her satirical sights on a culture of 'brave' and 'manly' collective repression (25), whilst upholding her own sentimental fiction as means of overcoming it.

[381] Eaton, 'Little Nell,' 274.

[382] Ripley argues that the 'appeal' of *Cold Feet* lies in its capacity to switch seamlessly between the 'painfully truthful' and the 'completely daft'. The enduring popularity of the series owes much to the skill with which it has 'married these two elements', as viewers deeply affected by one scene are given the balm of 'therapeutic escape' in the next (Dunn, 'Hugging People,' in *Cancer Tales*, 51).

[383] Schwalbe also draws attention to the value of escapist fiction for someone living with cancer, describing how reading fictional novels allowed him and his mother 'to simply be a mother and son entering new worlds together', an affordance Schwalbe explains that 'we both craved, amidst the chaos and upheaval' caused by his mother's cancer. See *End of Your Life Book Club*, 30-31.

[384] Dunn, *Cancer Tales*, 54-56.

[385] Eaton, 'Little Nell,' 275. The need for this form of 'holiday' is also underlined in an affecting scene in *Stepmom*, in which Jackie calls her young son from hospital, having just – unbeknown to her family – begun a course of chemotherapy. Trying to explain why she can't see her son for their regular Thursday evening treat, without revealing the truth of her situation, Jackie suggests they can 'meet somewhere special in our dreams'. Together, the two of them share a sentimental flight of fancy in which they visit a beach together. This

imaginative 'holiday' is meaningful for Jackie, shown tearful and alone in her patient's gown, yet her son struggles to understand why his mother is so invested in their game of make-believe: 'you don't need sunblock, it's a dream!' (68-69 mins). The scene might afford insights for family members or carers seeking to understand the complex emotional needs of a cancer patient, especially the desire to 'escape' their situation at certain moments.

[386] Deshazer, *Fractured Borders*, 150.

[387] Solomon, *Defense of Sentimentality*, 163-64.

[388] Deshazer, *Fractured Borders*, 150.

[389] Bouma and Ullestad, introduction to *Cancer and Theology*, xiv.

[390] Silver, *What Helped Me*, 182. These parallels in language suggest that Berg is evoking a sense of the 'open and ongoing spiritual search' that is a notable feature of the 'progressive spirituality' that has emerged in contemporary Western society in recent decades. See Lynch, *The New Spirituality*, 24.

[391] See Chapter 2, 57.

[392] Morgan, *Visual Piety*, 31.

[393] 'Love in small particulars' is the phrase used by Rowan Williams to capture the christological significance of Alyosha Karamazov's attentive, generous love for the minutiae of human existence. Alyosha's practical, grounded commitment to such love provides the counterpoint to Kolya's cold, absurd anti-sentimentalism, offering an alternative approach to the problem of sentimentality. See Williams, *Dostoevsky*, 36; and Ewan Bowlby, 'Theology, Cancer and Sentimentality in the Arts,' *Transpositions*, March 9, 2018, http://www.transpositions.co.uk/theology-cancer-and-sentimentality-in-the-arts/.

[394] Hopps, 'Introduction,' 23.

[395] Lynch, 'Role of Popular Music,' 486.

[396] Reybrouck, 'Musical Sense-Making,' 395.

[397] Hughes, 'Cold Feet.'

[398] The Kirkus review of A. J. Betts' teen cancer-romance novel *Zac and Mia* (Boston: Houghton Mifflin Harcourt, 2014), describes romantic cancer-fiction as a 'burgeoning subgenre'. Betts' novel plays on the tensions between the approaches of two teenagers diagnosed with cancer. Whilst Zac prefers to use the rationality of 'logic and math' to interpret his situation and chances of survival, Mia's response to

cancer is 'whipped up by emotion and impulse'. These contrasting styles afford interesting insights into the subjective, personal nature of an individual's reaction to cancer, as well as the false dichotomy set up between intellect and emotion. Patients tending towards either of these extremes might find the gradual intertwining of the two perspectives revealing. See 'Zac and Mia,' review of *Zac and Mia*, Kirkus, July 1, 2014, https://www.kirkusreviews.com/book-reviews/j-betts/zac-and-mia/. Other examples within this subgenre include Nicholas Spark's novel *A Walk to Remember* (London: Sphere, 2013), Jessie Andrews's *Me, Earl and the Dying Girl* (New York: Abrams Books, 2012), and Wendy Wunder's *The Probability of Miracles* (London: Razorbill, 2011).

[399] As well as paying attention to the responses of individual viewers or readers, it is tempting to suggest that all scholars commenting on the morality or spiritual value of a 'tear-jerker' should ensure that they are familiar with the genre and provide examples from specific artworks when they outline their criticisms.

Final Thoughts

[400] George Eliot, *Middlemarch* (Oxford: Oxford University Press, 2019), 125.

[401] Alistair Appleby, John Swinton, Ian Bradbury and Philip Wilson, 'GPs and Spiritual Care: Signed Up or Souled Out? A Quantitative Analysis of GP Trainers' Understanding and Application of the Concept of Spirituality,' *Education for Primary Care* 29, no. 6 (November 2018): 367-75.

[402] Fitch and Bartlett, 'Patient Perspectives,' 17.

[403] Frank, *Wounded Storyteller*, 11.